Grieving Mental Illness

A Guide for Patients and Their Caregivers

Second Edition

This is a self-help book for anyone who has endured the effects of mental illness, whether as sufferer, friend, family member, or caregiver. It offers detailed, jargon-free guidelines to help readers come to terms with mental illness in a positive way, while avoiding disabling emotional responses. Sophisticated in its approach and comprehensive in its treatment, *Grieving Mental Illness* will be useful both to health care workers and to the general public.

Virginia Lafond's experience as a mental health practitioner has taught her that grieving is always a partner to mental illness. Unacknowledged grief takes its toll, slowing or even stalling recovery. Using grief as a healthy, normal, adaptive process enhances recovery, allowing positive choices to be made. The result can help sufferers come to terms with their illness and prepare them for success in rehabilitation programs.

This second edition contains a new introduction and two new appendices: 'A Practitioner's Guide for Working with the Grief of Mental Illness,' and 'Grieving Mental Illness: Responses to Frequently Asked Questions.'

VIRGINIA LAFOND is a social worker in the Schizophrenia Program of the Royal Ottawa Hospital.

Grieving Mental Illness

A Guide for Patients and Their Caregivers

SECOND EDITION

VIRGINIA LAFOND

UNIVERSITY OF TORONTO PRESS
Toronto Buffalo London

© University of Toronto Press Incorporated 2002
Toronto Buffalo London
Printed in Canada

ISBN 0-8020-8532-6

∞

Printed on acid-free paper

National Library of Canada Cataloguing in Publication

Lafond, Virginia
    Grieving mental illness : a guide for patients and their caregivers /
    Virginia Lafond. – 2nd ed.

    Includes bibliographical references and index.
    ISBN 0-8020-8532-6

    1. Mental illness.   2. Grief therapy.   I. Title.

    RC455.4.L67L33 2002   362.2   C2002-903317-9

The University of Toronto Press acknowledges the financial assistance to its publishing program of the Canada Council for the Arts and the Ontario Arts Council.

University of Toronto Press acknowledges the financial support for its publishing activities of the Government of Canada through the Book Publishing Industry Development Program (BPIDP).

With gratitude to and in memory of

my mother, Louise Charlebois Johnsen,
who once even came to see me dance,

and

my father, Andrew Johnsen,
who also never failed to encourage me.

Contents

Foreword

Most of us recognize, when someone contracts a serious physical illness, that common reactions to grief – denial, anger, sadness, despair – are experienced, not only by the person directly affected but also by their family members, and, from time to time, by their professional caregivers. To date, however, we have not paid much attention to the occurrence of these same grief reactions in the face of mental illness. For patients this may be because the very symptoms of mental illness blur with the grief – for example, when they are told about their psychiatric diagnosis and the treatment involved. At such times, family members are concerned about discovering the best treatments for their loved ones, and aren't often aware of their own grief reactions. Professionals who treat mental illness also often fail to acknowledge and deal with the grief experienced by patients, family members, and themselves.

We could say that the entire history of mental illness is replete with denial – denial that such illnesses exist, denial that those affected by these illnesses have needs extending beyond their particular pathology (for example, adequate housing, decent income, fair work opportunities), and denial that people are emotionally and psychologically affected when mental illness enters their lives.

In *Grieving Mental Illness*, Virginia Lafond reaches beyond the illness itself and talks about the subjective experience that accompanies it – that is, what the *inner person* experiences when mental illness becomes a part of life's realities. She considers grieving with respect to mental illness as normal adaptive reaction. As well, she explains how the grieving process, though it does not heal the illness, can be used to heal the person affected by the mental illness experience.

This, however, is much more than a self-help book. It offers an important theoretical marriage – a marriage that joins the acknowledgment of what mental illness means to the person with an educational model for understanding and using the grief that accompanies mental illness. The offspring of the marriage is a developmental model of grieving, a model that shows how grieving can be a lifeline when mental illness enters our lives. In practice, Virginia Lafond's model will assist professional caregivers to understand that, because of the grief reaction, some of our educational efforts with patients and their families may sometimes fall on deaf ears. Furthermore, patients, family members, and professional caregivers will learn to view themselves and others more accurately and more sensitively.

Overall, *Grieving Mental Illness* gives us new grounding for practical and genuine empathy.

Barry D. Jones, MDCM, FRCP(C)
Chief, Schizophrenia Branch
Institute of Mental Health Research
Ottawa

Preface

This book has been written for those who suffer mental illness first hand, and for those who give care. It is based in part on the work I have done over the past several years with patients and their care-givers – families, friends, and professionals. It also springs from my own experience with mental illness.

My experience as a mental health practitioner has taught me many lessons. Chief among these is the understanding that grief, with its attendant feelings of doubt, sadness, anger, guilt, fear, and shame, is an inevitable partner to mental illness. Another is that grief's presence in these circumstances is rarely acknowledged by anyone.

The bottom line is this: those of us whose lives have been touched by mental illness have something to grieve about, and we need to get on with the business of doing that.

This book is meant to help you discover your own grieving process as a way of coming to terms with your mental illness experience. I hope it will also be a useful road map and guide for fellow travellers on the journey to recovery.

Acknowledgments

As I wrote *Grieving Mental Illness*, I frequently thought with a keen sense of gratitude about the many people who have influenced me, and, in a real sense, brought me to the point of writing a book – a point, by the way, that I still find somewhat astonishing. I wondered how one ever expresses adequate thanks. At this moment, I realize that saying *Thanks very much* is what is possible, and I trust that by saying so, the depth of my gratitude is to some extent conveyed.

First, special thanks must go to each of you who attended the Discharge Planning and Coping with Illness group sessions with me over the last eight years. Our valuable discussions made it clear that the link between grieving and the mental illness experience is basic to learning how to cope with the ravages brought by mental illness – and to recovering (or discovering) a sense of self. Outside the group sessions, your feedback affirming my efforts gave me the confidence to give a number of presentations and workshops.

I also want to offer sincere thanks to the many dedicated and courageous care-giving family members with whom I have worked. Whether I have met with you in our family information groups or individually, I count you as collaborators, but also among the best of my teachers.

I owe a special debt of gratitude to 'my friendly editors,' each of whom was kind enough to read earlier drafts of this book: Carol

Steinberg and Jo Weston (close colleagues in social work); Dr. Hany Bissada (psychiatrist and first-rate debater); Sisters Patricia Brennan and Patricia Jean Mulcahy (teachers, now retired, who haven't lost the knack for constructive criticism); Lyn Williams-Keeler (a colleague whose expertise in the field of post-traumatic stress disorder provided particularly relevant points of reference and departure); Chuck Spicer (chaplain and colleague, whose enthusiasm for this book was a great encouragement to me); Bruce, Sandra, Sheila, and Jodi (who know first hand the losses that come with mental illness, and who told me the book was worth reading); Alice and John (close, dedicated relatives of persons with mental illness, who also affirmed my work). Thanks so much for your careful and caring suggestions.

Special thanks to my colleague and friend, Susan Chiarelli, who listened, commented, and in other wonderful ways provided encouragement as I plodded through the writing. Your approval of a near-final draft was a genuine treasure.

Sincere thanks to Janet Joyce, chief librarian at the Royal Ottawa Hospital, for your ready and skilful help with my various searches through the literature.

Thank you, Joanne Haddad, instructor of psychiatric rehabilitation, for being the first to suggest 'spreading the word' about working with the grief of mental illness to promote recovery and to enhance rehabilitation.

I will always be grateful to Dr. Jay Weston, whose generous and wise counsel was always so tastefully and respectfully given at just the right moments.

Very special thanks to Dr. Barry Jones (chief of the schizophrenia program at the Royal Ottawa Hospital) who has always supported and encouraged my ways of working with patients and their families. Many thanks, too, for volunteering to be my 'agent.'

I would like also to extend thanks to the University of Toronto Press for accepting Grieving Mental Illness for publication. I owe special gratitude to Virgil D. Duff, executive editor, whose support for carrying the book forward was most encouraging.

Thanks and deep gratitude go to my family, especially my daugh-

ters, Louise and Simone, my sisters, my aunts, and my in-laws –
everyone who gave their wholehearted support for this venture.

Finally, a very special thank you to my husband, Raymond,
whose dispassionate, critical comments were almost always right,
and whose support was, as always, limitless. Thank you *mon
amour*, for everything.

Introduction

> Mental illness really takes its toll on our lives. In my case, I've lost my marriage, and my career – I was once earning fifty thousand dollars a year. Mental illness leaves us feeling we have lost control over our lives. Sometimes we don't know which way to turn. There's a real journey in coming to terms with this illness and its many losses.

Dan's[1] statement, though full of reasons for feeling sorrow, gave me a moment of contentment. Dan was stating openly what needs to be talked about, but isn't: people whose lives are shattered by mental illness have a lot to grieve about.

The grieving begins with the loss of health that mental illness is of itself, and goes on to include other major losses that can touch every aspect of life, both for those who suffer mental illness first hand and for those who give care.

As a professional caregiver, I have worked with people who suffer mental illness, and with their families and friends. I have witnessed and been touched deeply by the grief of mental illness: the shock, disbelief, anger, guilt, heartache, outrage, and, for many, the disappointment that the illness they are experiencing cannot be cured, only treated. Often there is also self-doubt and self-blame: 'Did we cause this? Where did we go wrong?' There is anger at the profes-

---

1 The names of persons quoted or referred to in other ways are fictitious. To respect confidentiality, some biographical details have also been changed.

sionals: 'Doctors should have medication for this.' There is struggle: 'My husband has an illness that makes his behaviour terrible to live with, but I feel that to leave him would be to abandon the love of my life.' There is shame: 'I've behaved so weirdly when I've been really ill, I've shamed my children and my husband forever.'

Especially early on in our experience with mental illness, feelings and thoughts take second place to concerns about medications, other treatments, and expected outcomes. Later, however, loaded down with unresolved grief, we feel exhausted (sometimes frankly ill) from dealing with the experience whether we suffer it ourselves or are caring for someone who is ill. Failure to recognize mental illness as loss and to do the necessary 'grief work' takes its toll.

> When grief is looked upon as a valid and, in its own right, interesting topic of study, it becomes possible to treat it in a way that neither trivializes it nor puffs it up; to treat it, in effect, as another part of the life-space which must be examined, understood, and assimilated ... Willingness to look at the problems of grief and grieving instead of turning away from them is the key to successful grief work in the sufferer, the helper, the planner, and the research worker.[2]

Colin Murray Parkes, eminent pioneer in the field of grieving, demonstrates through his research that there are similarities in the way people, over time, come to cope with different losses. These similarities form patterns which show that 'stages' or 'phases' are present in the grieving process. Because of his work and that of other grief theorists, notably Elisabeth Kübler-Ross, denial, sadness, anger, and acceptance are concepts many are familiar with. Indeed, countless numbers have found this knowledge helpful when dealing with events commonly recognized as losses: the death of a loved one, the amputation of a limb, the destruction of one's home. This information forms a large part of the foundation on which this book stands.

---

2 Colin Murray Parkes, *Bereavement: Studies of Grief in Adult Life*, New York: International Universities Press, 1972.

There is no doubt in my mind that these concepts are of immense value to those of us who experience grief because of an encounter with mental illness. Perhaps most enlightening *and* comforting is the knowledge that the grieving process has stages or phases, including one of acceptance. Also, specific information about these stages can give us some needed light, not only 'at the end of the tunnel' but also for use on our journey. If we allow ourselves to have some faith in what the grieving experts tell us, I believe we can experience some easing of our pain.

If you have doubts about using the grieving process to come to terms with your mental illness experience, let me assure you that you have lots of company. Actually, I have found most people to be cautious until I explain the following two basic points:

1. The process of grieving mental illness *is* a positive experience through which hope can be rekindled.

2. Renewed hope gives each of us a chance to make other positive choices for ourselves.

From the outset it is essential to appreciate grieving as the healthy, normal, adaptive process it is. As you proceed through this book, you will see that grieving becomes effective when we give ourselves permission to become *conscious* of what is happening to us, and to both *tune into* and *work with* that process. As we move from unconscious grieving – being unaware of how we are feeling – to engaging in the grieving process consciously, we enable and enhance our recovery from our mental illness experience.

Consciously grieving mental illness can bring healing to many, even all, aspects of our lives. It can help us become aware of the coping skills we already have and how to use them better. It can also help us develop new ways of coping, reduce stress, and boost our self-esteem. For those who suffer mental illness first hand, the conscious grieving of mental illness could help you prepare, not only for a formal rehabilitation program but also for your ultimate success in such a program. For family members, friends, and other caregivers, having a better understanding of the links between loss, grieving, and mental illness can help you use your grief to come to peaceful terms with your experience with mental illness. Finding some peace in the midst of the mental illness maelstrom is absolutely essential!

You will notice throughout this book that phrases such as 'the mental illness experience' are used rather than simply 'mental illness.' This has been done for two reasons: (1) to emphasize that *Grieving Mental Illness* is not only for those who have first hand experience (patients), but is also for anyone whose life has been touched by mental illness; and (2) to make it clear that this book does not focus on healing mental illness itself; rather, it is about ways and means of coming to terms with – indeed, recovering from – the effects of mental illness on your life and particularly on you as a person. In other words, while healing mental illness would refer to treating its symptoms (so that acute episodes of mood swings, hallucinations, delusions, and depression are resolved), *Grieving Mental Illness* deals with healing the emotional and psychological wounds that occur as a result of the mental illness experience.

Because the conscious grieving process is essentially a journey, *Grieving Mental Illness* is meant to be a road map for that journey. Scattered throughout are a number of signposts that highlight key points to shed light on your path. You will also find several exercises especially developed to facilitate the process of conscious grieving. In Chapter 1 we will explore the dynamics of the grieving process and learn what must be done to begin grief work. The second chapter deals with coming to appreciate mental illness as loss – loss that inevitably triggers other losses. In four of the last five chapters we will look at the different stages or phases of the grieving process (denial, sadness, anger, and acceptance) and learn how these can be 'worked' to bring about recovery. Chapter 6 is devoted to dealing with that powerful feeling of fear, which I see pervading the whole grieving process as it relates to mental illness.

You will also find in this book examples taken from real life stories, including my own. My personal experience of recovering from the impact of mental illness took literally years, following as it did a very uncertain course. I didn't have a road map!

Before beginning writing I struggled to decide whether or not to disclose pieces of my own psychiatric illness history. I was concerned about conveying a kind of 'I've done it so you can too' message. While I believe that kind of message can be useful in some self-help books, I believe it is almost at cross-purposes with my reasons for writing this one. First of all, I respect the fact that each person's journey in coming to terms with the experience of mental illness as a *unique journey.* Also, I am well aware of the different kinds of impact mental illness can have on each individual affected, whether he or she suffers them first hand or experiences them 'secondarily' as a caregiver.

Thus, I want to emphasize that I chose to share parts of my experience for only two reasons. First, when I look back on my journey to recovery, I remember that whenever someone who appeared to be well told me about their personal struggles with mental illness, I felt less alone. These were priceless moments for me – moments that are precious to this day. Second, as I have worked and learned as a professional in the mental health field, I have drawn on my experience as a psychiatric patient. Initially I drew on this experience rather reluctantly, and certainly always in the secret place of my own head. However, gradually I came to see that my combined experiences as a psychiatric patient and a mental health practitioner put me in a rather special position. Eventually, with the encouragement of some close colleagues, I was able to acknowledge that my psychiatric illness experience, even the most painful and embarrassing moments of it, was a valuable resource. From this resource I learned profound lessons. Over time, I have incorporated these lessons into my work in an attempt to assist others – those who suffer mental illness and their caregivers – to come to terms with the consequences of mental illness. Their feedback – that working consciously with the grief of mental illness is genuinely helpful – has given me both permission and the courage to illustrate some points in this book with one of my best conscious grieving process teachers: my own personal mental illness experience.

I now believe that the stages or phases of grieving can be psychological and emotional landmarks, maps, and keys to recovery from experiences with mental illness. However we choose to think about them, we know they are there. Each of them offers its own challenges to every one of us, patients and caregivers alike. We can all begin, begin again, continue, or approach the finish line of our grieving journeys.

My wish for each of you, as you read and use this book, is that you find peace.

Introduction to the Second Edition

On occasion over the last few years, I've recalled my many moments of trepidation as I wrote *Grieving Mental Illness: A Guide for Patients and Their Caregivers*. These feelings arose as I recognized that my ideas would come across as new, and perhaps startling, to many (though I knew that I hadn't invented notions about grief in connection with mental illness), and because I was keenly aware that I was putting these ideas together for people who were suffering. I wondered if my articulation of ideas would make sense and, even more, be genuinely helpful to my audience. I most certainly wanted to do no harm.

I worried also because my writing – at least in part – drew on my own mental illness recovery experience, and would therefore be perceived to be on academically shaky ground. I managed, however, to reassure myself. It was, after all, my experience of being left in a state of emotional and psychological confusion once the symptoms of my mental illness had abated, along with my later professional experience of working with people on a psychiatric ward, that prompted my first questions in the area of the grief experience. Thus, for me an important question to be answered was, 'How do we help people deal with the psychological and emotional consequences of the experience of mental illness?'

Since *Grieving Mental Illness* was first published in 1994, I have been, to say the least, very pleased with its success. I've also been pleased to receive from readers a good number of descriptions of how exactly the book has been of help.

Some of the comments caught me by surprise. Family members pressed the point that the book's message gave them something new – permission to grieve the experience of mental illness as it touched the lives of their loved ones as well as their own lives. As one mother put it, 'Since I read your book, I know that I don't always have to grin and bear it. I can still be a caring mother and cry about this – even openly at times.'

People affected first-hand expressed two reactions. First, that I knew what I was writing about, and second, that learning that their feelings about having to deal with mental illness were normal helped them to feel respectful of themselves and not so alone. I've been delighted to hear words to the effect that the book helped them to be kinder to themselves as they've walked the recovery journey.

It's been gratifying to hear people talk about embracing their grieving process and going with it – consciously and constructively – and coming to a point of integrating the experience of mental illness meaningfully into their lives. Or when people remark that, rather than sinking into what they thought was another bout of depression, they've instead recognized their grieving and used tools suggested in *Grieving Mental Illness* – and have found themselves not only avoiding depression but seeking and reaching a new level of recovery.

I've also found myself blessed to hear from colleagues who work in various branches of the mental health field (addictions, children's services, geriatrics, and forensic psychiatry) that *Grieving Mental Illness* gave them new and valuable tools, or reinforced the grief work they were already doing with patients and their families.

In addition to providing positive, affirming comments, readers have also asked a good number of questions and offered some criticisms, including the surprising comment that grief is the 'wrong metaphor' for what happens to people as they process the experience of mental illness in their lives. These I've accepted as gifts, ones that have over time helped me to improve and further develop my ideas about work with the grief of mental illness.

The publication of a new edition of *Grieving Mental Illness* provides a timely opportunity to respond *en masse* to the most frequently asked questions, many of which have come from workers in the mental health field. In this volume you will find, in Appendix I, a practitioner's guide to working with the grief of mental illness, and, in Appendix II, responses to six questions I've been asked in the course of facilitating workshops and making presentations since the book was first published. I hope that both appendices will be valuable additions.

Finally, I wish to offer my profound thanks to everyone who ever invited me to speak, asked a question, or made a comment about work with the grief of mental illness. Without your participation, I would likely still be feeling those lonely moments of trepidation I felt in the early 1990s. I also give thanks to my life partner, Raymond Lafond, who read several drafts of the material for this new edition and made many good suggestions. As well, I offer heartfelt thanks to University of Toronto Press for publishing *Grieving Mental Illness* in the first place, seeing it through two reprints, and now issuing this new edition. In particular, I owe Virgil Duff, my editor at University of Toronto Press, very special thanks.

Virginia Lafond, MSW, RSW
9 December, 2001

Grieving Mental Illness

A Guide for
Patients and Their Caregivers

ONE

Learning to Work with the Grieving Process

'I feel lots of negatives but I think overall I can just say, I hurt.'

'I feel cheated. I think I'm mostly feeling angry.'

'I've disappointed my parents. This makes me sad.'

'I'm scared. I feel I'm never going to get well again.'

'My overall feeling about my husband's illness? We've both suffered tremendous losses. I know I'm still hurting, even though it's been years now since its onset.'

Each of these statements indicates the speaker's awareness of a predominant grieving feeling. When I'm working with people who are dealing with the effects of mental illness in their lives, I recognize statements like these as milestones, and, in a way, as cause for celebration. Why? Because when people put names to the negative feelings they experience because of mental illness, they have claimed ownership of those feelings and can then do something with or about them to promote personal recovery.

Before this, not knowing just exactly what our feelings were, together with their sheer weight, made it impossible to call the feelings by name and speak clearly about them.

Coming to an ability to name and claim our feelings shows what is called 'process' at work. In other words, we are gaining the ground we need to take control of our lives and are in a position to do something with and about our feelings.

In this chapter, we are going to look at the basics of grieving. Specifically, we will explore the meaning of process, the role of awareness, the dynamics of the grieving process, and the important differences between *unconscious* and *conscious* grieving. We will also focus on an outstanding grieving problem for both patients and their caregivers: grieving a loss when it is not recognized by society as loss.

SIGNPOST: *Awareness of what is happening within ourselves makes a world of difference as to how we live our lives*

Process, whether psychological, spiritual, emotional, or physical, always implies motion. Its opposite is stagnation and stillness – a state of being 'stuck.' Human beings, like all living things, are always in process. Sometimes we are very aware of our processes, but often we are not. However, when we consciously tune in to what is happening emotionally within ourselves, we are in a position to choose to make certain uses of our feelings. For example, we can decide in the face of a sad event that it is perfectly appropriate to seek out a friend and cry on his or her shoulder. Or, when something good happens we know we have reason to rejoice and will act accordingly: phone our good news home, say, or throw a party.

Actually, while journeying to recovery from our various encounters with mental illness, using awareness of our process is essential. And, it is important for us to know that we *can learn to use* it as a trusty guide – one that will help us know when to stay put, when to move on, when to try something new, when to take a break.

SIGNPOST: *To learn to grieve consciously we must decide to do so*

In order for awareness to function at its optimal level, we must give our consent. In other words, we must be willing to cooperate with it in helpful ways. It is, in fact, our *willingness to be aware of our grieving process that makes the crucial difference between unconscious and conscious grieving*.

Think about the following statements. They show very well the difference between someone who is grieving but is not aware of the grieving process, and someone who is aware and is grieving *consciously*.

'Feel? I couldn't tell you how I feel. Maybe down. Anyway, I don't care how I feel. What's it to you?'

'I know I'm in a kind of mourning because my daughter has a chronic mental illness. I get really down about this sometimes, and when I do, I try to do something for myself ... to bring at least some relief to the weight of the feeling. Otherwise I get overwhelmed.'

Conscious grieving is a decisive act, one that requires an act of the will. We cannot drift through it or simply let it happen. This is a journey we *choose* to make, and every step of the way we must be alert as we actively, gently, and firmly work towards recovery.

You see, the process of grieving *does* go on whether we are conscious of it or not, so we might just as well decide to *use the already present process of grieving to help us progress*. This is like taking the driver's seat of an already moving vehicle. Just as the driver of a car has decisions to make while on the road, we have decisions to make in the 'vehicle' of our conscious grieving process.

When we have climbed into the driver's seat of this vehicle, determined to *make it work* for our recovery, we can and should take heart. Clearly, when we make this choice we have taken ownership of our grieving process, making rehabilitation and recovery possible.

SIGNPOST: Basic points about grieving

Let's look at some important information about the phases of grieving: denial, sadness, anger, and acceptance.

• Feelings at each stage of the grieving process can all be felt at once, and often are. There is nothing abnormal about having mixed or even confused feelings. Often, though, one particular feeling can be recognized because it is felt more strongly than others.

• Once you have passed through various phases of the grieving process and feel you are in an acceptance stage (where, at least, you are able to note that you are feeling more peaceful), don't be alarmed if, suddenly or gradually, you feel renewed sadness, anger, or even denial. *This is perfectly normal.* As human beings, our internal processes are always complex, sometimes wonderful but often painfully unpredictable. We need to learn to remind ourselves that a myriad of internal and external cues are at work, stimulating different aspects of ourselves – including our powers of memory. And when painful memories return, our more painful grieving reactions can again be felt (and, sometimes, strongly). However, if you have been engaged in your grieving process in a *conscious way*, there are these blessings:

• You know you have made it through before.

• You now know you have the skills to cope with grief.

• Most of all you know that, though it will take effort, you *can cope with and use* the returning feelings of grief.

The *only* feature about grieving considered a problem is staying 'forever' in an early grieving stage.

SIGNPOST: Problems arise because ours is unrecognized loss

> We who have adult children who are mentally ill are not understood. People in general do not know what we go through. What hurts most is when my own sister and brother either turn deaf ears to us or criticize whatever we do for our son. In their opinion we're either doing too much or too little ... I am convinced that no one really understands the agony we go through.'

Agnes's words point out vividly the additional problems faced by those who suffer loss when there is no formal recognition of that loss by society. These problems do not usually occur when, for example, we grieve the death of a family member, because a death in the family is an event society recognizes as loss. When someone close dies, friends and family gather and enter into various established grieving rituals: funeral arrangements are made, cards of condolence sent, and prayer services and wakes held. And someone often stays with the bereaved for a time after the formal services. These rituals provide spaces for talk, tears, and even laughter. When there is a death, we *expect* grieving and we support each other as we grieve.

As Agnes's words indicate, this is far from the response encountered when we are grieving the losses that mental illness brings. Agnes and her husband not only have to experience their grief without the support of close family members, but also in the face of their criticism.

Another problem is that *even we* who are faced with the losses associated with mental illness often do not 'register' these events as losses. This lack of acknowledgment is a significant roadblock to our coming in tune with the grieving process; for example, when we tell ourselves we shouldn't cry when crying would be in fact one of the most healthy, appropriate actions to take.

To take away some of the sting we feel when our losses go unrecognized, it is helpful both to identify these problems and to have some understanding as to why they occur.

SIGNPOST: Look for 'no room for grieving' messages

> I go to a psychiatrist for myself. She knows my daughter has schizophrenia but she won't let me get into that. She won't let me cry about it. She's told me to come back when I'm ready to get on with things.

Help with grieving the losses of mental illness often cannot be found, even in places we might expect it – that is, where mental illness is treated. Rarely will psychiatrists or other mental health practitioners talk to their patients or their patients' family members about the experience of loss related to mental illness. To some extent, this is understandable, given that doctors and other health professionals are not specialists in grief counselling. Even if they have such training, they often fail to see mental illness as a subject for grief work. In some cases, when illness can be treated but not cured (as in is the case of major mental illness), professionals can sometimes see this outcome as their personal failure. In practice, the primary focus of mental health professionals is treating *the illness in individuals*, but they do not usually recognize or treat the illness *as loss*.

Where does that leave us? Certainly, with a number of challenges, the first of which must be to make a decision to take responsibility for finding our own way through the grieving process. It is important to note here that I am not suggesting 'going it alone.' An *essential* part of finding one's own way is finding companions for the grieving journey.

I have come to see that there are some major advantages in having to find one's own way. I discovered this by accident when I was trying to recover from one of my bouts of mental illness. During this time, I had had several check-up visits with my physician. At different points during these visits, I tried to express how distressed I was because I now had a 'psychiatric patient' label. He never once responded to what I was saying about this, but instead changed the subject. At the time, I interpreted his lack of acknowledgment as a message that I was speaking about an irrelevant, unimportant, 'shouldn't-be-bothered-with' subject. Years later, I came to the realization that my doctor either could not deal with aspects of my grief about my mental illness experience, or he did not see it as falling within the realm of his work with me. Those check-ups provided me with my first lessons about how professional helpers can be *unhelpful* in addressing with their patients some very real and troubling aspects of having mental illness (e.g., living with a label). For me this was the beginning of many lessons, one of which is that, though we expect something different, individual professional helpers often provide a limited range of service.

Where does this leave us when we have needs that lie outside the realm of a professional helper's practice? In short, we are left with the job of looking elsewhere for the help we need. By doing so, we take ownership and responsibility for our recovery. We start to become *active players* in our recovery process.

How do we behave as active players in our own recovery? For one thing, we stop saying simply, 'Yes, Doctor,' and start saying, 'Okay, Doctor, you have explained that treatment and I now have a pretty good idea about its pros and cons. You have also answered my questions. *I have decided* to go along with your advice.'

When we begin to make decisions for ourselves, we take giant strides away from feelings of powerlessness ('Everybody tells me what to do. Everybody but me is in charge of my life.'), and we start to feel in control.

Another important point: We must be prepared to feel lonely. Grieving in relation to the experience of mental illness is a lonely experience – yes, sometimes even when the support of relatives, friends, and other caregivers is present. Still, we do need others. And I want to be perfectly clear about this: taking charge of our lives does not mean getting rid of doctors, nurses, social workers, and other professional helpers. On the contrary, it means *working with them* on our own behalf.

So far we have learned that grief is a process, and that awareness of our grieving process and consenting to work with it are critically important for recovery from the mental illness experience. We also know that the impact of mental illness is not readily recognized as loss – as a subject for grieving. Finally, we see that our recovery from loss starts when we take charge of our own journeys, including finding sympathetic and appropriate helpers along the way.

TWO

Grieving Begins with Acknowledging Loss

In this chapter we will look at the immediate troubling consequences of mental illness: the side effects of medication, the cost of treatment, the changes in income, and the reactions of family, friends, and colleagues. Though all of these problems can be classified as losses, very few of us would stick a 'loss' label on them. Instead, most of us would label them 'problems to be solved.'

Grieving experts tell us it is not surprising that we fail to recognize mental illness as loss at the early stages of its entry into our lives. In fact, as we will see in the following chapter, denial of loss is a normal part of the grieving process. But the grief experts also believe it is important to *come to recognize* our experience with mental illness as *loss to be grieved*. Here, at this point on our journey to recovery, it is vitally important to emphasize this point once again.

You see, if we fail to call what has happened to us loss, we can begin to lose touch with the healthy parts of our lives or forget to give ourselves credit for them. Possibly, too, we won't use them. Remember, rarely is anyone mentally ill *through and through*! Rarely is life completely void of normalcy, of happy aspects. But life can appear totally bleak if we don't do some loss/non-loss stocktaking.

SIGNPOST: *Grieving can put us in tune with the healthy side of ourselves*

It is very common for people facing mental illness to feel psychologically paralysed, confused, dispirited, in broken-hearted pain, and totally absorbed by its impact. For example, consider the parents who have just seen their son off to college, only to receive a call from a psychiatrist a few months later telling them their son is in a psychotic state. At this point, the parents would naturally focus on what is wrong and how it can quickly be put right. They will ask questions about the seriousness of their son's condition, how long it can be expected to last, what treatments are available, and which treatment the psychiatrist is planning to use.

Similarly, when a woman who has recently given birth is told that she has a problem in the psychiatric realm,[1] and that she must be hospitalized, her attention would most surely be on getting answers to her questions about when she can expect to be 'back to normal' and just how she's going to get there so that she can take care of her baby.

If the young man's condition subsides, but flares up again, and if the mother does not get better within the time she expects to, *then*, and usually not before then, the patients and families may begin to look at how the mental illness experience means loss for them, and how other losses have come into their lives because of it.

SIGNPOST: When we see mental illness as loss we are at the starting point of the conscious grieving process

How do we get a sense of the losses brought into our lives by mental illness? Usually, my answers to patients are slightly different from those I give caregivers. I recommend to patients that they start by identifying the aspects of themselves affected by mental illness (their moods, thoughts, abilities), and then evaluate these to see what the consequences have been. For caregivers, I suggest they consider that their loss involves not only how the mental illness has affected a member of their family, friend, or patient (client), but

---

1 This is likely the way she would be told. People who suffer mental illness (and their families) are often not told the name of their illness clearly. At the onset of mental illness, this is usually related to uncertainty in the psychiatrist's mind about the exact diagnosis. Later, not knowing or comprehending the psychiatric label often leads to failures in communication between the psychiatrist, the patient, and the patient's family. (Questions aren't asked; clear answers aren't given.)

also what unhappy outcomes it has brought to them. In other words, everyone touched in some way by mental illness needs to look at what the illness has done and is doing to bring unwanted and unanticipated changes to their lives.

At this point, with the *conscious* grieving process initiated, we should remind ourselves again that we are engaging in a normal, healthy process – that is, we are using our healthy, reactive, adaptive mechanisms. And, as we do this, we are also enhancing our efforts if we tell ourselves that it is *because we are aware* of the presence of the grieving process that we can *make greater use of this awareness* to help ourselves heal. As you proceed on your journey, also keep in mind that, *if we allow it*, healthy conscious grieving will help us get in touch with and use other healthy aspects of ourselves.

Making these conscious efforts may seem less than second nature at first. As one person put it, 'Thinking about what I'm feeling? Usually I just feel my feelings and think my thoughts!' Right! Usually, we do not stop to think about which aspects of ourselves (moods, thoughts, feelings) or our lives (relationships, job, residence) are healthy, which are affected by illness, and which may have marks of both health and illness. Because this kind of analysis isn't part of our 'thinking routine,' we are not up-and-ready, that is, in the position to use our healthy side to compensate for and cope with what is problematic, painful, and unhealthy. But we can learn. In fact, learning new ways of seeing and doing things is now the task at hand.

SIGNPOST: We can change the way we see

The three exercises that follow have been designed to assist you as you begin working in a conscious way with your grieving process. I urge you to take whatever time necessary to put yourself through the paces of these exercises, and to repeat them whenever you feel the need to do so.

EXERCISE 1:

It is often helpful to begin the grieving experience by looking at circumstances other than our own. Take the next few minutes to get a sense of the loss contained in the words of three people who have encountered mental illness. Try to avoid getting into a problem-solving stance by thinking of solutions. Simply attempt to capture and feel the aspects of loss in each story. You will be experiencing their loss at those points where you would want to offer sympathy.

'I was at university when I first got sick. I was planning to be a computer programmer. Though I've tried to start up my studies again I haven't been successful. A career as a computer programmer is no longer part of my plans. Now I have no plans.'

'Before I crashed with this, whatever it is, I could easily predict what I would do in a day, a week, a month. In fact, I'd make plans for myself and my family – you know, arrange schedules and things. Since I had my break, I'm never sure anymore if I'll feel well enough to carry through any plans, or to have enough motivation even to get started on a certain day.'

'My son was always on the go ... active in everything: sports, student council, out with his friends, at his part-time job as a waiter. Now he's completely changed. Always at home, unless we've cajoled him into coming out with us. Rarely, and I mean rarely, does he do anything on his own ... except to smoke cigarettes and watch television.'

These accounts give us obvious reasons to pause and feel sorry about what has happened to these people. We find we take into consideration:

• The former student's feelings of loss regarding her ability to be a student, the loss of confidence in herself, the loss of her way of life (her routine, friends, the joy of completing assignments, parties), the loss of her future (her career hopes, her income expectations). Granted, nothing was written in stone before, but she did have plans. The absence of these plans is loss.

• The disappointment of this mother, realizing that she has lost confidence in her ability to plan family activities. As well, she knows that she can't rely on feeling well enough to participate in any plans she does make. She hardly recognizes herself since her encounter with mental illness. She misses her former confident, energetic self with whom she has lost contact.

• This parent speaks about his son with a bewilderment still present even though the onset of illness occurred five years ago. He can hardly believe that the chain smoker in front of the TV is the same person who was once so full of spunk and promise.

Remember, these accounts are meant to heighten your ability to appreciate loss. As you read them again, try to curb any tendencies to think about cheering the father on to see the healthy aspects of his son, or helping the would-be computer programmer reduce her stress enough to return to school. Simply concentrate on the *sense of loss* in each story. It may help to

• Imagine the changes in each one's day-to-day life.

• Notice your reactions and the reactions you anticipate from others (any traces of stigma? a sense of failure? feelings such as 'this can't be true; somebody's got to be exaggerating?')

• Get a sense of any other feelings of pain, such as sorrow, guilt, or anger.

EXERCISE 2:

The purpose of this exercise is to ensure, as much as possible, that you are convinced that the efforts you are now making towards your recovery, through the conscious use of your grieving process, are normal and healthy – that, in fact, you are using the healthy side of you to bring about recovery. I suggest that you (1) pause to think about this, (2) meet any barriers which might at this point be cropping up, and (3) give yourself credit (this is *very* important!) for what you are doing now.

SIGNPOST: Grieving barriers can be removed

It is important that you take deliberate notice of any barriers you encounter and attempt to take charge of doing something about them. Two common road-blocks to normal grieving are well-intentioned but problematic advice from others ('Get your mind off yourself. Your problem is that you're dwelling on your problems!'), and your own unconstructive self-talk ('It's selfish to think about myself. I shouldn't be dwelling on myself.').

Rather than let these barriers take charge of you, find your own words (or use mine to begin with) and say loudly and clearly to the barrier, 'I am attempting to get well. I have been told that the first step is to be in conscious touch with how much my (his/her) psychiatric illness has hurt me.'

If you have never taken a moment to face what mental illness has meant to you, congratulate yourself for doing so now. You have begun the process of conscious grieving. Even if, some time ago, you started to grieve your experience with mental illness *consciously*, tell yourself you are doing well. This is an important affirming message to give yourself.

It is essential that you give yourself pats on the back, and use other ways to support yourself throughout this conscious grieving journey. You know that through your experience with mental illness you have met huge challenges. You know these can touch all aspects of life. So don't downplay what has happened to you in any way. Mental illness has left you in pain, in fear, in shock, without confidence, with feelings of hopelessness and powerlessness. Though with time the intensity does lessen, the feelings do not go away. And because they are present, they can and most probably do still affect you. Therefore, you need to give yourself all the affirmation and support you can find: friendly, constructive self-talk, pats on the back, hugs, and other rewards.

If you feel ready, move on to Exercise 3. If not, take and enjoy a break of whatever length you need, and then do Exercise 3.

EXERCISE 3:

When you first attempt conscious acknowledgment of the losses that accompany mental illness, you may feel little emotion or you may feel a whole range of emotions. Most people report having a mixture of painful feelings – feelings they often have difficulty naming. What is important at this stage is not that you can or cannot find labels for these feelings, but that you are making an effort to 'get at them' – that is, to reach for them and attempt to feel them fully, or at least as fully as you can. The more you practise feeling your feelings, the easier it will be for you to distinguish one feeling from the other. As mentioned earlier, once you can name your feelings, you are in a position to own them *or* disown them as you choose.

The major purpose of Exercise 3 is to introduce you to the skill of asking yourself the two basic and most important questions of the conscious grieving process:

1. How can I help myself cope with _____ ?

2. Are there ways I can use my experience of _____ constructively?

The blanks in these questions can be filled in with particular feelings (sadness, frustration, fear, anger) or with specific circumstances (difficulties in family, professional, or other relationships; money problems; the illness getting out of control again).

The first question is *the* key coping question. It is to be asked whenever you encounter a negative feeling or circumstance in relation to your mental illness experience. Have it ready (I mean as ready as a carpenter has nails and a hammer), ask it, and look for answers. You may find that satisfactory answers come to you easily by simply being open to asking the questions. Undoubtedly, though, there will be times when you will need to seek out someone you trust to help you figure out realistic, helpful ways of coping. Once again, I emphasize the importance of doing this. Remember, grieving is always hard. We need others.

In the group work I do with patients, whenever someone talks about feeling sad, angry, or bothered in some way, we ask, 'How do you help yourself cope with your *sad/angry* feelings?' Answers can often be found by looking at what we have done in the past to alleviate negative feelings. The answers that come – taking a walk in the fresh air, talking about the problem, watching a baseball game on television, having a warm bath with a book in hand (one of my favourites) – are all ways of coping successfully, of doing something about our burdens.

We know these coping skills have worked for us before, and there is no reason not to use them again and again and again! Best of all, these tried-and-true remedies remind us that we have the power within ourselves to help ourselves.

Once we have been through this exercise a few times, most of us come to recognize that we have a whole range of coping skills (though granted, we haven't been used to calling them coping skills). Often, too, some of them have to be brought out of mothballs and then freshened because we have kept them, unused, in storage. Learning to acknowledge and use coping skills for the specific purpose of making life easier is of utmost importance. One significant bonus is that we are not only making life easier but we are also rebuilding, at the same time, an essential ingredient for our health and well-being: self-esteem.

Now to the second coping question: Are there ways I can use my experience of _____ constructively? *Using the experience of a feeling constructively* means that we identify the energy that is part of any feeling and put this energy to work. *Using the experience of a circumstance constructively* means identifying what we have learned from a problem situation or event and using that knowledge for our own or another's benefit.

In the conscious grieving process it is critical that we *become comfortable with our uncomfortable feelings*, so that we can allow ourselves to be in intimate connection with this aspect of our healthy selves, and can learn to use these feelings as the energy resource they are.

Here is an account of a family member who has obviously learned to help herself cope with uncomfortable feelings, and to put what she has learned to constructive use:

> I knew my anger and my sorrow were justified when he became really ill again. And I knew that we would all be on an emotional roller-coaster as we faced what would unfold during and after this episode. However, this time I wasn't telling myself to keep a stiff upper lip. I found that, in deciding to let myself cry when I felt like it, and to feel my anger, that I was not fighting myself. I wasn't giving myself all the 'You should do this' messages I once did. I found I was coming to a true sense of respect for myself. My life was much easier.
>
> Learning that it's healthy to feel my feelings has not only been personally liberating. I have also learned from this experience the importance of respecting others, even when our feelings and opinions (theirs and mine) are different. I can see that I've put my feelings to good use.

If you feel ready to put your feeling or experience to good use, ask yourself for specific suggestions about how to use the feeling or experience. Make sure your answers are realizable – timewise, moneywise, and energywise!

In the following chapters you'll find several examples for rebuilding coping skills, starting with the basic feelings experienced in grieving. For now, I would suggest that you follow through on the suggestions that come to you *as long as they are not hurtful to yourself or those around you.* Try to get into whatever you do wholeheartedly. Whenever you make attempts to concentrate, for example, on a game you have chosen to play or watch, be assured that you will make gains. Remember, there are always gains to be made when we devote our entire attention to an activity. Emotional and intellectual diversion, and thus relief, are part and parcel of our efforts to recover.

SIGNPOST: Focus to name feelings accurately

When you were doing the first two exercises you were employing a skill called focusing – a skill that enables us to single out our problems and the feelings we have about them. We can also use focusing to test out our negative feelings, to see if there is an appropriate fit between them and to see what is happening in our lives. Focusing is a particularly valuable skill to use when guilt (a very common experience in the lives of patients and their caregivers) creeps in.

Joan's experience with guilt during a period of hospitalization shows how focusing can work. Married with two children, Joan stated that she was feeling a lot of guilt:

> I feel I should be at home helping my son with his homework instead of spending evenings on the ward socializing with other patients. And my husband now has at least a double workload ... and he takes time to come and visit me. I've put burdens on everybody!

When I suggested that Joan attempt the coping skill of focusing to determine what the basis of her guilt feeling was, she quickly answered that it was simply 'plain guilt.' But once she began to examine this feeling, looking for a *reasonable fit* between her guilt and being sick and in hospital, she realized there was no clear reason to feel guilty. After all, she had done nothing *morally wrong* by coming into hospital. She had not *caused* the chemical imbalance that underlay her mental illness.

I urged Joan to continue her efforts at focusing in order to discover what she was feeling. With further effort, she concluded that her overall feeling was one of sadness. This feeling felt 'right.' She missed her children, and the day-to-day routine she and her husband had established for themselves. Having recognized what her true feeling was, Joan now felt entitled to feel 'down' about landing in hospital again.

At this point, I suggested that she ask the key coping question: 'How can I help myself cope with my sadness?' I suggested she look back and see how she had successfully coped on previous occasions when she had felt sad. Joan's response was not unusual. She told me she often found that talking about her problems helped, as did having a good cry. 'Talking and crying,' she added, 'don't exactly *solve* my problems, but after I do feel like some of the weight of the feeling leaves me and I feel things will get better. I'm a little more hopeful.'

SIGNPOST: A few precautions as the journey continues

1. When you are about to do one of the suggested exercises, it is very important to find yourself a safe place. A safe place is one that both physically and psychologically provides a comfortable, quiet, calm haven that is, as much as possible, away from distractions. Your seat on a crowded bus or subway may give you lots of time, but not the privacy and silence you need and deserve. Tell yourself that you merit the closest thing there is to a gentle relaxing atmosphere, and take the steps to find this for yourself.

2. When engaging consciously in the process of grieving mental illness, be sure that you make a deliberate effort to respect yourself. Remember that one of your aims is *to recover* or *to discover* what is commonly called a sense of self. You will be working against yourself if, in getting in touch with your feelings and working with them, you also get into any kind of mental browbeating.

I suggest two commandments for this journey:

- You shall appreciate your experience in all its aspects.

- You shall give yourself a healthy dose of benefit of the doubt, especially when you find you are being hard on yourself.

3. When we attempt to remember how we have managed bad times successfully in the past, it often happens that fresh feelings of pain and disappointment rise to the surface. For example, people can feel that they will never again be anywhere near as successful (peaceful, contented, etc.) in the future as they were in the past. This kind of thinking can lead us to hopelessness and helplessness.

If you are feeling hopeless, focus on doing the best you can for yourself in the present moment. Open yourself to allowing time, therapy (medication, counselling, etc.), and the support of friends and relatives to do some healing – even if you have been through this many times before. It is important to keep in mind that *though you may think you will never regain your previous level of ability or your former peacefulness, you do not know that for sure.* Many have found, when they have reached a rock-bottom low, that this is the point where they have encountered new hope for themselves, including new ways of seeing and doing things.

4. As we noted before, it can happen in therapeutic sessions that the therapist will fail to affirm your losses related to mental illness. If your therapist does not allow you to vent your feelings, but instead wants you to look at ways to problem-solve or concentrate on the positives in your life, you may find yourself short-changed. You might even get the idea that dwelling on your losses is inappropriate and to be avoided.

It is a good idea just to be aware that mental health practitioners who work in institutions (whether hospitals or community centres) are likely required to work within institutional guidelines. Because these guidelines may limit services, practitioners will be looking at ways to solve problems as soon as possible. This, combined with the lack of recognition that mental illness means loss, will often work to stifle the attempts you make to get help with grieving your mental illness experience in those quarters. Watch for this! Seek out at least one person, professional or otherwise, who understands the benefits of the normal grieving process and who is willing *to be with you* while you dwell for awhile on how and why you are hurting.

In this chapter, we acknowledged that mental illness is a loss, one that brings other losses into our lives. We began working with our grief in a conscious way. We saw that a safe place for grief work is both necessary and what we deserve. We learned that measures to build self-esteem are necessary for making the journey to recovery. Next, we will examine in detail the role played by the denial stage of the grieving process, and how denial relates to the mental illness experience.

THREE

Denial Doesn't Deserve Its Bad Reputation

Up to this point, we have covered some basics about the grieving process. We have also looked at mental illness and seen it, not simply as illness but as loss. And we have seen that mental illness brings with it a host of other losses.

Now we are prepared for a careful look at each stage of the grieving process so that we will come to understand:

• what happens in each stage or phase;

• how we can use the experiences of each stage, not only to ease our pain but to promote our recovery.

Denial is often described as the first stage of grief, and, of all our grieving reactions, it is undoubtedly the most misunderstood and maligned. The following are just a few examples of wrong ideas about denial:

'She should be past denial. After all, she's had this illness for years now.'

'For such a bright person, he sure hasn't got much insight!'

'My son seems to want to stay in denial.'

Each of these statements shows that the speakers do not understand how denial operates, and, more important, that they do not see *it can and does serve a healthy purpose*. First, denial essentially has nothing to do with the length of time mental illness has been present, and it has little if anything to do with a person's level of intelligence. The last statement is simply a judgment call, born of the pain of seeing that one's adult child is not recovering as expected. It is based on the mistaken notion that being in or out of denial is a matter of will.

SIGNPOST: We are in denial because we need to be in denial

Denial, like the other grief processes, is not something we choose to experience. It happens spontaneously to help us cope with the reality of mental illness, just as it does when someone close to us dies or when we experience any other major loss. Like the other stages of the grieving process, denial is normal and healthy. Like sadness and anger, denial can become unhealthy *only* when it lasts too long. And what is considered too long will differ from one person to the other. We all march to our own interior drummers as we move through the stages or phases of grieving.

Most often denial kicks in immediately or shortly after a loss is experienced. It allows us to take in only bits and pieces of information about our loss as we struggle with our readiness to face the experience more fully. In other words, denial protects us from being crushed by the brute force of the reality of our loss.

Family members and professional caregivers hear a range of denial expressions from those who suffer mental illness directly:

'I'm not sick. You're sick!'

'I don't need medication. I just need rest.'

'The people who brought me here are out to get me.'

'I don't need to be here.'

'All I need is just a place to live.'

My experiences as both a professional caregiver and a psychiatric patient have helped me understand the three major ways denial works in people who suffer mental illness first hand:

1. People suffering mental illness are not trying to be difficult, resistant to treatment, or stubbornly 'in denial.' They simply *are* in denial. Besides realizing their loss of mental health to some degree, or recognizing that *something* is *radically different* for them, each one is having to grapple with other losses: admission to a psychiatric facility, the label 'mental patient,' being required to stay with others who are behaving strangely, a job lost or jeopardized. It is precisely because the experience of mental illness is heavy – too heavy to be taken in all at once – that denial comes into play. Denial puts a protective coating on the message about the illness and the other losses the illness brings. It clouds it up, making news such as, 'You are suffering mental illness' less real and thus less painful. For caregivers, a terribly frustrating but common result of this distortion of the facts by denial is that the people they care about will argue in various ways (including rude and crude ways) that they do not need help.

2. For caregivers, both family members and professionals, hearing messages of denial is also a 'loss experience' for themselves. Anyone trying to assist someone in desperate need of help will be affected when that person refuses the help offered. As a caregiver, I experience feelings of sadness and frustration when I attempt to work with people who are in denial and in obvious need of help. Understanding how and why our human mechanism of denial works has helped to increase my empathy for the person wrestling with information about illness – information that is always hard to hear. I think caregivers need to appreciate that we speak a *message of loss* each time we say something like the following:

'You need to stay in hospital for the next few weeks.'

'We think you need the help of a psychiatrist.'

'You can't live with us until you get psychiatric treatment.'

'This medication will help you.'

When we see that we are speaking a message of loss, we will at the same time know that the person to whom we are speaking will be assisted in absorbing this message by denying it.

3. For those who suffer mental illness first hand, denial often has unhelpful companions.

When a loss such as a sudden death of a loved one occurs, most of us experience a normal 'It can't be true' kind of denial, followed by the absorption, albeit painful, of the reality of the loss. For the person who experiences mental illness, the healthy denial process is often not as simple (if simple is ever a word we can use when speaking about a loss experience). Unfortunately, for the sufferer, denial is usually 'fortified' by the mental illness. Schizophrenia and the affective (mood) disorders, for example, often make taking in and using information extremely difficult.[1] Because of the ways some types of mental illness work, all messages, including those meant to be therapeutic or helpful, can become garbled in their meaning. As well, frequently enough, even someone close to the person suffering illness can appear as an enemy. Also, the person suffering mental illness often feels a decline in concentration ability.

These difficulties, *added to denial*, often have caregivers in despair: 'He'll never take medication!' 'My mother won't hear of going to a psychiatrist – she never has and never will.'

Well, maybe they won't ever change, but *maybe*, and I'd rather say *probably*, they will. The fact is that you and I do not know. As a professional helper, I accept as an obligation that I must live in hope that people will find their way. I cannot give up on someone because that person has not so far shown any acknowledgment that she or he has mental illness.

When I look back on my own psychiatric illness experience and look for clues indicating denial, I have difficulty finding them.

1 I do not mean that people with chronic mental illness (like an affective disorder or schizophrenia) have a constant level of difficulty in comprehending information. However, the way some mental illnesses work in waves or episodes can make for severe periodic difficulties in many areas, including that of understanding information.

There is no doubt, of course, that during my first round of illness, both the illness and the denial process were working powerfully to reinforce each other. The word 'denial' would not have been part of my vocabulary at that time because I knew nothing about the stages or phases of the grieving process. Nor did I have even vague knowledge about the consequences of the mental illness experience on oneself and on others.

My 'world' at that time was full of threats, guns, and bugging devices (the latter a sign of how greatly my psyche had been influenced by the then current Watergate news). I remember also that for a period while in hospital I was convinced I was going to be shot by a hired gun, aimed and ready in the window of a nearby apartment. As I interpreted things at the time, anyone who tried to persuade me otherwise just didn't understand the reality and urgency of my situation. (To this day, I'm grateful that my fear was taken seriously – my insistence that my husband stay with me that night for my protection was accommodated.)

No doubt, I was 'in psychosis.' Though I can now see that my ways of perceiving, thinking, and doing then were clearly coloured by both denial and illness, I know that try as my caregivers did to convince me that there was no danger, I wasn't always able to change my mind to their well-meaning, realistic points of view.

At other times I was able to comprehend and agree with the reality of what was said. I also felt terribly discouraged when I realized the seriousness of my mental illness. However, at these same moments I began to ask questions important to my recovery, questions such as, 'What do I have to do to get out of hospital?' I also remember making mental notes to avoid talking out loud about ideas I knew would seem crazy or inappropriate to others. Doing this helped me regain my ability to make judgments about my own behaviour, including what I talked about.

As I look back on my journey through illness, I can see that I first rejected various caregivers' points of view, and later used many of them as points of reference. To my caregivers, I know that I often appeared to be very much in denial, in psychosis, or both. But I know that their points of view, especially when expressed with care and respect, played an essential part in my recovery.

SIGNPOST: We work through denial in our own individual way

One of the reasons I have described this part of my own illness and recovery process is to encourage caregivers who may be giving up hope. Don't give up. Just know that everyone's experience is different. To get well, some of us need to hear different people say over and over that the illness affecting us is a real problem that needs and deserves treatment. For others, denial seems to abate only when the force of the illness abates. Still others only experience insight into their illness through tough trial-and-error methods – for example, by discontinuing treatment only to find themselves hospitalized again.

Just remember that messages from caregivers are more likely to be heard if they are given in easy-to-understand, firm, and *gentle* language, and if they are not loaded down with detail.

SIGNPOST: Caregivers can help when someone is in denial

As caregivers, I believe we must keep trying to influence the person who is in denial about their mental illness experience – if for no other reason than to give them some relief. Now, I am not recommending that we argue with people until they 'get the message,' or try to 'hammer our message in.' I am recommending, however, that caregivers do speak clearly and assertively to patients from time to time about their illness and its consequences.

Make your points in ways you know won't lead to endless debate or hurt feelings. For example, it is often helpful to:

• Keep statements short and clear.

• Remember, you are not trying to win your point but to assist the person you care about.

• Keep all remarks free of blame.

• Whenever possible, choose a quiet, calm, non-threatening atmosphere to make your points.

• Give persons suffering illness respect whenever they hold views different from yours.

SIGNPOST: *Caregivers deserve a respectful hearing, too*

If you are suffering mental illness first hand, I suggest that you ask this question: 'What do my caregivers need or deserve from me as they try to help me move through denial and other phases of my grieving and illness process?'

Wearing both my psychiatric patient and professional helper hats, my suggestions are:

• Show openness and a willingness to hear what is being said.

• Respect the message, even though you might not be in agreement with it.

A capacity for openness is often only possible in the denial stage for those who have suffered *more than one* bout of mental illness. In most cases, patients recognize only with hindsight that denial was at work, or, as in my case, only when they are consciously looking for evidence of it.

It took me a long time to recognize how denial affected my course of recovery. My denial mechanism was undoubtedly bolstered by at least two of my personality traits: I don't have *unquestioning* openness to the opinions of others and I can be fairly easily irked by probing questions. For example, I remember that I was very annoyed with my husband when he kept asking me questions I thought were ridiculous. When he asked if I remembered where I had parked the car, I felt like telling him to mind his own business, though I knew that I couldn't have told him where the car was. What did that matter? I thought. There were more important things to talk about at that moment. I also resented his comments about my sleeping habits. So what if I got up and walked to the post office at 5:30 a.m.? And wasn't it perfectly okay to take a bath at 2:30 a.m.? 'There's nothing wrong with me,' I remember telling him. 'I just have loads of energy.'

Of course, as I look back, I can see that there *was* something wrong. The fact was, I couldn't get myself organized to accomplish tasks that at other times I would have done easily. Basic housekeeping ceased to be important. To this day, I shudder with embarrassment to think of the room I provided for a favourite aunt who had come thousands of kilometres for a rare visit. Though I knew of her visit well in advance, I didn't lift a finger to change the condition of the guest room, which we were then using for storage. Because illness *and* denial were very active in my life at the time, things like laundry, meals, guest rooms, and other household matters were often badly neglected.

SIGNPOST: Denial and illness are not blameworthy, they are opportunities for learning

When patients (and caregivers) look back on their denial phase, they can tend to blame themselves for being in denial. For a long time after I recovered, I was convinced I should have been able to come to grips with my illness and its consequences sooner than I did. Actually, throughout my first bout with mental illness, I was deeply bothered by the idea that my illness shouldn't be happening to me. My thoughts alternated between 'You're too grown up for this to be happening' and 'If only you would use your intelligence, you could get well!' Many years later, when I had become familiar with grieving process theory and felt safe enough to look at what I could recall about my own denial stage, I *finally* gained some valuable insights about myself. Only then did I begin in earnest to accept my illness experience.

I still feel some embarrassment when I think about things I said and did in the denial stages, but hindsight, together with knowledge of denial's purpose, has shown me that I needed to be in denial *precisely because my illness was traumatic and its wound was too intense to be felt all at once.*

When I hear patients apologizing or showing feelings of discomfort such as embarrassment, shame, or guilt, I hear a need for more education about the denial stage of the grieving process. Here's an example of what I say to assist people to understand denial and how it helps us adapt to our serious losses:

> Denial operates like a shock absorber. When we have seen television reports of major catastrophic events, usually there is evidence of shock shown by eyewitnesses. They may be tearful, talking rapidly, or barely able to talk, or they may in fact appear stunned.
>
> Trauma theory experts indicate that what is reported by witnesses often differs from 'the facts.' The witnesses didn't lie. When their ability to absorb and process the disaster information went into gear, a kind of built-in safety net (often called shock reaction) was deployed. Because of this, some bits and pieces of information were perfectly clear while others were missing or confused.
>
> If an event is bad enough some will say, 'It can't be true!' or 'I don't believe it!' What has happened is that the objective facts of the catastrophe were as they were, *but* the denial mechanisms within each of the witnesses went into operation to allow them *to absorb the information in a healthy, adaptive way*, each according to his or her own built-in readiness sensor.
>
> Later, these witnesses usually have other normal reactions: they may lose sleep, their eating habits may change, or they may find themselves 'numb,' dwelling on different painful aspects of the incident, or fighting to put them out of their minds. Whatever the reaction, the shock absorption process is normal and healthy. Denial, one of the most essential features of absorbing painful information, is *normal*.

SIGNPOST: How do we know we are in denial?

I'm always glad when group members ask whether they could be in denial and not know it. It gives me the opportunity to make these three points:

1. Simply because you are open enough to ask that question, it sounds as though you are well on your way out of or past denial.

2. There are aspects of every stage of grieving which will always be with us, because whether we grieve consciously or unconsciously, we never completely lose our sense of the loss. This sense – the

heavy, painful, wretchedness – may cause fleeting or even more lengthy returns to denial.

3. *If* you suspect you are hampered by denial, you can use the key question for building coping skills – in this case, 'How can I help myself with my denial?'

In group work, answers to that question nearly always include suggestions *to ask* questions and *to get* understandable answers about diagnosis, treatments, expected outcomes, and rehabilitation programs. Remember, we always have a right to any information about ourselves. Rather than seeing our appointments with mental health professionals as one-sided examinations or treatments, we can use them as opportunities for negotiating about ourselves.

If you believe you are hampered by some remnants of the denial phase of grieving and feel you are ready to deal with them, try the following exercise. Its purpose is to help you feel more comfortable about the past by seeing it in clearer, fuller context.

EXERCISE 4:

Proceed through this exercise with the advice of one of my mentors in mind: 'Take a *gentle* look at whatever bothers you.' Get a sense of exactly what is still bothering you by recalling details of the particular experience – where it happened, who was involved, what was said, what you think others felt, what you felt. Remind yourself that you are not recalling this memory to depress yourself, but only to help yourself evaluate anew what it is about the situation that you had, and are still having, to deal with. Ask yourself if there is anything you can do now to resolve this matter. If the situation, for example, involved someone you can approach now, perhaps discussing the matter with that person will alleviate the problem for you. If you judge that there is a good possibility this could be the case, take that course of action. If not, make a decision to let it go. This problem is hampering you. Events we can do nothing about always need to be surrendered eventually, so that we can move on.

The importance of respecting yourself throughout this exercise cannot be emphasized enough, because this exercise can be painful (pain we usually try to avoid by avoiding exercises like this one). Who wouldn't want to forget running naked through the neighbourhood, making dozens of long-distance phone calls (and the bill for them), or punching someone while being 'out of control?' Similarly, most of us would rather forget what doctors have told us about our psychiatric problems or the mental illness being experienced by someone we care about. None of us wants to hear, for example, that schizophrenia is an incurable condition that requires medication for an indefinite period. Or we don't want to hear that our judgment is impaired, especially when we believe other people, including the doctors, are wrong and meddling in our lives.

As you, at your own pace, go about the business of consciously thinking about your experience with denial and mental illness, you will probably notice other feelings, such as anger, sadness, or fear as well. It is *always* important to recognize that these feelings are normal and healthy reactions to the impact of mental illness. This recognition that our painful reactions are part and parcel of normal living is a step towards appreciating them as valuable in the healing journey. Openness to our feelings, being purposely and wilfully in touch with our emotional selves, is an essential part of becoming whole and remaining as healthy as possible.

Initially, you may baulk at suggestions that you become comfortable with your feelings. As we know by now, *feeling* our feelings is not always easy. This is not only because feelings can be painful, but also because of the many insensitive remarks we encounter about normal human expression of emotion. Sometimes we even hear them from professional caregivers. I once heard a professional comment after a talk a man had given about the illness and death of his son. It was her strong opinion that the man should deal with his 'unresolved emotions' before giving further talks. Is it any wonder we find ourselves in the position of having to learn how to welcome our emotions, claim them, and use them for our benefit?

I suggest that you repeat Exercise 4 as often as it is of help to you. By repeating it, you will build insight into your experience, an invaluable tool for keeping yourself on the path of recovery.

In this chapter, we have dislodged some mistaken ideas about denial and have looked at how and why denial works *for our benefit*. As we continue to progress, our awareness will lead us to other stages of grieving. Next, we will examine the role sadness plays in our recovery journey.

FOUR

Be Sad!

We receive constant messages from our cultural environment about how to feel and when to feel. These messages work with a powerful, yet usually unrecognized, force against experiencing feelings such as sadness. 'There's no sense crying over spilt milk' is the type of adage that can wield tremendous power in many areas of our lives, often to the extent that it works against our normal reactions to life's harshest circumstances. As noted earlier, a shock-absorption mechanism is also at work to cushion the impact of our loss, and it kicks in to assist us with integrating our experience with mental illness. This denial mechanism, as we saw in Chapter 3, has other outstanding virtues. It can also hand us opportunities to break through its safety net so that we can begin to work with and on the feelings that, though hidden, are present nonetheless.

This chapter explores ways to undo some of the power of the sadness-blocking messages in our culture. It is also aimed at helping you recognize and use situations commonly encountered in the sadness phase of grieving, so that your recovery is not slowed down or halted by roadblocks.

At some point after the onset of psychiatric illness, and before the resolution stage of recovery (acceptance), feelings of sadness come both to those who directly suffer illness and to their caregivers. How people experience sadness depends to a large extent on individual circumstances. For those who have experienced major chronic illness in themselves or in others, the sadness (and other difficult emotions) can seem relentless. On the other hand, for those who have suffered one or two episodes of psychosis, have regained their health, and live apparently without any psychiatric-illness residue, the feelings of sadness may be more or less obscured. Feelings of relief that accompany what appears to be a full recovery may for some time mask feelings of sadness. This is wonderful for as long as it works, but experience has taught me that most people who experience a recovery like this live with a good deal of fear and other emotions simmering on the backburner.

Feelings which have not been tuned into, responded to, and used to enhance recovery, to *the person* can potentially influence literally everything a person thinks, does, or says. To illustrate, think about what would happen if we were to ride a ten-speed up a hill – in the wrong gear. If we were to do nothing about switching to the correct gear, the efforts we made to ride uphill would result at least in a pain in the legs, and chances are we wouldn't make it to the top.

SIGNPOST: It's normal not to know how you're feeling

Now, let's look at ways to get our feelings in gear so that we can avoid expending more energy than needed.

To begin, let's recall an important point: When we talk about sadness, or any one of the other feelings at play in the grieving process, it is essential to tell ourselves that it is *perfectly normal* not to have felt a certain feeling clearly enough to be able to name it. When most of us are asked how we feel or what we are feeling immediately following an unusual and traumatic event, we often answer something like this:

'I don't know.'

'I guess I'm feeling hard hit.'

'Feel sorry for myself? Maybe, but not much.'

'I'm happy it wasn't worse.'

Sometimes feelings of fear and anger can be overwhelming. At these times they often crowd out feelings of sadness, so that getting back in touch with our sadness can take a good deal of work.

Looking back on my own psychiatric experience, I know that 'I'm sad' would not have been my answer if somebody had asked me how I was feeling about having mental illness. Having had several years to think about names for my feelings in the early phases of my illness, I would probably describe them as stunned bewilderment or embarrassment. Certainly, I have since felt, and sometimes still feel, great sadness, both for myself and for those close to me when I think of the things that happened (and didn't happen) because of my illness. An example: The almost new condition of my second daughter's Baby Book will always be a sad testament to my withdrawal into illness. She and I will always be deprived of the joy of remembering her first tooth and when she took her first step. I now know that as painful as a recollection like this one is for me, there can be several advantages to feeling the pain. In feeling sadness about it I feel 'connected,' to myself and within myself. Another way of putting this is that I am both facing and experiencing my emotional reality.

SIGNPOST: It's normal to see-saw

See-sawing during the grieving process happens when the person goes up and down or back and forth from one grieving stage or phase to another. In my practice, I have often seen people who appear to be more angry than sad, then return to a state of anger, and later become noticeably sad again. The same thing can occur even after an acceptance (or resolution) stage has been reached – that is, when strong coping skills have been part of a person's repertoire for some time. As we noted in Chapter 1, if see-sawing occurs after the acceptance stage is reached, these skills, learned and honed during the process of consciously grieving, can be used to return to the more peaceful stage of acceptance. This return is usually – but not always – accomplished in less time than it took to get there at first. Asking the key coping questions ('How can I help myself cope with _____?' and 'Are there ways I can use my experience of _____ constructively?'), and following through on the answers that come, can prove to be of invaluable help in regaining personal control over see-saw motions in one's grieving process.

SIGNPOST: *What's not normal?*

The only things you need to watch for on your recovery journey are:

• staying in one stage of grieving for too long;

• staying on the see-saw 'forever.'

These two ways of experiencing grief are not only not helpful or useful, they are also seriously unhealthy. Whether you are a care-giver or a person who suffers mental illness first hand, these grief experiences often work to keep you emotionally stuck in a rut. They can literally lock the doors to your recovery. However, when you come to recognize that the grieving process is the companion of mental illness, and when you learn how to use it consciously, you will have the master keys to recovery in your hands.

SIGNPOST: *Facing your sadness brings relief*

Here is a simple, three-step formula for *using*, not just feeling, your sadness:

1. Tell yourself it's okay to feel sad.

2. Take time to *experience* sadness as an 'Okay feeling.'

3. *Use* sadness for recovery by asking the critical question: 'How can I help myself cope with this feeling?' and by putting your answers into action.

By telling ourselves it's okay to feel sad about how mental illness has affected us, we are giving ourselves huge lessons in self-acceptance and self-affirmation. We are also acknowledging that we understand the basics about living healthy, well-adjusted lives. We realize, if we have a particular feeling, that there are reasons for its presence. By paying attention to the feeling, we can check it out for its appropriateness – but not before we say to ourselves, 'It is *perfectly acceptable* for me to feel sorry for myself.'

Several 'healing pay-offs' happen when we stop saying, 'I know I must not feel sorry for myself' and move to saying something like, 'When I think about it, I do feel downright sorry this happened to me.' Some people report that, for the first time, they have taken their *selves* into account enough to notice their sadness. In group work, when I say that people often feel 'depressed about being depressed, but don't usually talk about that,' I have heard and seen many genuine, even enthusiastic, expressions of agreement. Immediately, but with shyness, people begin to talk about how painful their feelings of sadness are. Instead of talking about the wounds of their illness, they talk about what this wound has brought to them, including their sense of self-esteem.

It is at moments like these that healing begins in earnest. As we tell our stories of what we experienced, as we reveal *what really happened to us*, and as our stories are respectfully listened to, we often feel a sense of renewed hope. This new sense need not be of the one time, 'guest appearance' variety. Hope has staying power if we give ourselves permission to repeat the steps outlined above.

EXERCISE 5:

I encourage you now to find your own words to convince yourself that it is okay to be sad about your mental illness experience. Remember to find your safe, calm place and to quiet down and rest, breathing deeply and slowly. Talk to yourself supportively about the importance of realizing that you are entitled to feel sad about the losses you have encountered.

If you seem to be speaking a foreign language, be assured that you probably *are*. This kind of self-talk *will* be foreign to you. Just tell yourself that you must keep talking like this in order to destroy the old negative messages. If left unchecked, those old 'It's bad to feel sorry for myself' messages will again get the upper hand. If you have difficulty with this kind of supportive self-talk at first, persevere. With practice it will not only begin to make sense but will become second nature.

SIGNPOST: Feeling sorry for yourself has its benefits

When we have given ourselves the green light to feel sorry for 'me' we can begin to take inventory of everything that has happened to us throughout our experience with psychiatric illness. By counting our losses and giving them a thorough appraisal, three things happen:

1. Sad feelings take on a shape.
Most of us can see that there is a 'fit' in the degree and quality of our feelings and our losses. When we discover this fit, we know it *is* okay to feel sorry for ourselves.

I can hear the critics: 'Don't people tend to exaggerate and wallow in self-pity?' My answer to this is a firm 'No.' Most people, given the chance to talk about their losses and their feelings about their losses, do so with words that show they are groping for clarity. As they become comfortable, feelings are described with increasing precision. What may be interpreted as wallowing means, more often than not, that they are in the very necessary phase of feeling the pain. It is only when this pain is felt and appreciated, at least to the extent that the feeling is recognized, viewed as appropriate, and literally 'suffered,' that a person can make conscious choices about this expression of sadness.

2. We 'get our act together.'
Parts of ourselves, alienated so much that we hardly recognized them as our own, are brought home. Feelings that we knew only vaguely are now not only allowed to be experienced but also can be put to work through the act of consciously grieving them. When we are sad and we know it *and* are showing it, we are basically acting in healthy, truly *wholesome* ways.

3. Decision-making becomes the agenda.
We have decisions to make about the sad feelings – which need not
be a frightening prospect. If you have tuned into yourself, for example, by accepting the feelings you have stored in some distant part
of yourself, you have already taken significant steps towards being
in control of your life. Remember that you are working, through
conscious grieving, to become your own driver. Your 'chauffeurs'
may still be in your employ, but they will be getting directions from
you.

SIGNPOST: You have a mountain of choices

As one of my professors was fond of reminding us: 'There are only
three things in life we *have* to do: eat, sleep, and excrete – all the
rest are *choices*!'

As we saw in a previous chapter, conscious grieving, by raising
our awareness of what has happened and what is happening to us,
brings with it the opportunity to make choices. Some wise soul
once likened grieving to peeling off the layers of an onion. As we
peel, the onion's scent stings our eyes and we cry. But once we have
closed our eyes and wiped away the tears, we can decide either to
stop peeling the onion, take a break, or go on peeling the onion.

You will discover layers of choice on your journey to recovery
when you ask the first key question of the conscious grieving process: '*How can I help myself cope with* _____?' Whether you fill the
blank with 'my feelings of sadness,' 'my fear of returning to work,'
or 'my lack of hope for a return of my son's health,' you have set
out to find opportunities for making decisions – and they will be
there! At the same time you are showing yourself that you can find
your own way – a way that *fits you and your particular needs.*
Decision-making with your well-being in the forefront can, and
usually does, work to change longstanding feelings of being
trapped by circumstances.

I have some suggestions that relate to choices to be made, and I
will get to them shortly. First, please take note that no one can or
should be trying to make choices for you as you experience your
sadness. Some people will always try to tell us what we *should* be

doing (and, to be fair, it may be their way of showing they care). We also tend to give ourselves plenty of 'I should' messages. Not that there is anything intrinsically wrong with the word 'should,' but its indiscriminate and frequent use is growth-preventing and a definite block to recovery.

A rule for handling all 'should' messages is to hear them as suggestions rather than commands. In other words, use them as points of reference to consider as you decide what actions to take. Many people report great changes (some call it growth) within themselves once they learn to hear commands as suggestions. They say they are no longer being pushed by 'shoulds' and are breathing the fresh air that comes with making their own decisions.

The moment I recaptured a sense of control of my life stands out on my list of personally significant turning-points: My husband and I were driving to a movie, when, very caringly but firmly, he began to give me directions about an application I was making to graduate school. (In other words, he was telling me what I *should* do.) As I listened, I realized I didn't agree with his advice. Deliberately formulating my reply, I said, 'My benevolent dictator, I hear what you're saying and I appreciate the care and love that's in it, but the specifics don't feel comfortable to me at this point, so I won't be taking your advice. My plan is to submit my application the way I have judged it to be right for me.'

Believe me, that was a giant leap! I had made up my mind about how I was going to do my own business, despite my partner's reasonable counsel. The postscript to this story: I have subsequently made several more decisions in the same way and my marriage has not fallen apart. If anything, it has matured and continues to bloom.

SIGNPOST: Try tempering your sadness

1. Cultivate your sense of humour.
In my experience, very few people display a robust sense of humour, whether they are sick or well. People who encounter mental illness do tend to take *everything* seriously during certain phases of illness, and this is to be expected. Mental illness, especially in its

early stages (and sometimes in later stages), offers very little opportunity for joke-making or the enjoyment of lighter moments. What we can do in periods like these is *work* to make life a little easier through the use of some well-chosen humour (taking care not to use risky practical jokes). A cartoon on the jacket of a book on depression has the right spirit: A husband is saying to his wife, 'Another depression, dear? Let's make up our minds to enjoy this one!'

The idea is to do something! Take breaks. Feel the sadness and know it is okay, *but* know also that it is okay to distract yourself from it, to be frivolous and have fun.

EXERCISE 6:

Before you try this exercise, take a moment to evaluate your reaction to the material we have just covered in the last paragraph.

Did you hear my words as commands or as points of reference?

If you heard them as the points of reference I meant them to be, you are clearly on your way to taking control of your life – or you may have arrived at this point already. You have not left the control to others. Congratulations! This is achievement indeed.

If you heard my suggestions as commands, please remind yourself that you are entitled to take advice only if you want to – in other words, nobody passes or fails this exercise. Its main purpose is to help you gain a better sense of where you're at when it comes to assuming control in your life. Its second purpose is to emphasize that combining humour and sadness is not an impossible endeavour. We only learn to achieve a fitting balance of the two with practice – and plenty of it – which reminds me of that question, 'How do you get to Carnegie Hall?' and its answer: 'Practice! Practice! Practice!' (Just a suggestion, mind you!)

2. Don't travel the sadness road alone.
You may think you should not burden others, or perhaps you prefer to keep to yourself. Remember, human beings are social animals, with a basic need to relate to, with, and among others. The social part of ourselves does not dry up when we are grieving – if

anything, it is more present. As we saw earlier, many subtle (and not so subtle) messages from our culture (not being a burden, even to family, for example) would have us deny this. Granted, many people do buy into it. My point in mentioning these popular ways of thinking is to have you ask yourself if you want *these ideas* to *control the way you think*, or if you would rather challenge them in order to *do what feels right for you.*

If you do not feel motivated to exercise the 'social animal' side of yourself, try this: pick someone you have known to be understanding of you in the past. If you are worried about burdening this person, make the decision that you will not let that happen. Make up your mind, for example, that you will, with genuine interest, ask what is happening in your friend's life. Listen carefully, ask other questions, and comment on what he or she says in response to your questions. *Then* try talking about yourself. If you are still worried about burdening your friend, ask, 'Do you mind listening?'

At this point we sometimes encounter responses such as, 'I can't listen to you.' or 'I don't want to listen and I'm not going to,' or 'Let's not dwell on this. Here, I'll make you a cup of tea.' If this happens to you, move onward. Find somebody else. As one well-informed counsellor put it, 'Don't be on a friendship diet.' Remember, you open yourself to receiving the support you need and deserve once you attempt to eliminate your concern about being a burden to another.

If you have looked for and believe you have found a professional helper, that is well and good. If however, you are seeing a professional who doesn't seem to appreciate what you are trying to say, or if you find yourself saying, 'He doesn't seem to understand what I mean when I tell him _____' or 'She's telling me I shouldn't place so much importance on _____, but I still have this problem,' pay attention. Not every professional is comfortable with pain and tears. Remember, you have a right to choose a professional helper who will meet your needs.

SIGNPOST: Are you 'therapist-hopping?'

To avoid harming yourself, there is one point that requires careful attention. Some people move regularly and frequently from one professional helper to another, and they do so because they cannot or will not hear what the helpers are saying. If you believe this is true of you, try to examine what has been happening in your therapy. Are you avoiding an issue that calls for you to sort something out? More important, are you in danger of overdoing the therapy process and ending up with what is called an 'iatrogenic' condition – in this case, a condition caused by treatment from too many different professionals? If so, what's the remedy?

Begin by looking at your pattern of therapist-hopping. Then consider negotiating with your therapist to make the relationship more suitable to your needs. Simply making your needs clear, or clearer, can help immeasurably. You become more confident if your therapist knows clearly what you want from the therapeutic relationship. This is not always easily accomplished, but it is worth working on. If you are trying to become more assertive and you have a therapist you feel is not meeting your needs, I suggest you practise assertiveness with your therapist. You might just find that you have no need to move on.

If you still want to change therapists, discuss your intention to move with him or her (that is, the one you intend to depart from), whether you feel like it or not. Any helper worthy of the title will want to know why you are moving on. A 'closing conversation' with your therapist will also keep the relationship on honest terms, which leaves the door open for you to return if you choose to do so.

SIGNPOST: Learning to handle desperation and despair

There are many reasons not to isolate yourself when you feel sad, but the principal ones relate to the danger of slipping into helplessness and hopelessness. In the helping professions we often see people who are already wounded by their experience with mental illness being wounded again because they believe no one can help or no one cares. You may *believe* that this is your situation, but by choosing a conscious grieving route, the opportunity is yours to choose to think, and come to *believe*, that people care about you and can help. You *can* help yourself change your feelings of desperation and despair. As always, our *openness to change is key.*

The next exercise is designed to help you fine-tune your ideas about caring – giving it, using it, and depending on it.

EXERCISE 7:

This exercise is for people who are struggling with feelings that theirs is a hopeless situation and that no one can or is willing to help. It has two parts.

First, picture a person, someone other than yourself, hungry, homeless, and out in a storm. She is tired, cold, and penniless. For reasons of her own (she may be thinking for example, 'I've always been a private person.' 'I've been able to make my own way' ... 'They won't understand' ... 'They will blame me'). She does not bother the people in the homes around her. She has nowhere to go. She sits on the empty sidewalk and the tears come.

You are inside one of those homes. You are warm and well fed. What is your reaction as you consider this woman's plight? What do you feel you want to do? Take at least five minutes to think about your answer.

Most of us will find ourselves wanting to help this troubled woman. We may not know exactly how we can help her, but we do know that by leaving her alone we do no good at all. If we could, chances are that we would go to her, let her know that we are there, and that we care. What might happen next would be anyone's guess. She might say, 'Get lost!' She might say nothing. Or, she might tell her whole life's story or just a part of it. Who knows? The important thing is, you *are* there with her.

What do you want to do at this point? Perhaps you have questions to ask, such as 'How did you get here?' or 'Why are you here?' or 'Couldn't you _____?' But you *are there*. You are offering her much-needed companionship because you realize she at least needs your presence. You know, in your heart of hearts, that you want to be there for her.

In the second part of this exercise, you are the one feeling desperate to the point of hopelessness. Now imagine some good soul approaching you and offering to be there with you. Are you going to open up to this person or not? Or will you let your feelings and beliefs about yourself ('I am a private person' or 'Nobody can help me') win out? Or are you going to see the sense in letting someone be a crutch for you, at least for a while?

If you are about to decline this person's offer of help, review how *you* felt in the first scenario when you approached the destitute woman in the street. You wanted to help her, at least in some way, right? Even if you didn't have much time to spend with her and her problems, you still wanted to help her to feel better. Your feelings were genuine. You wished that her hope would be rekindled because she chose to see that your offer of help was sincere.

Our wishes for ourselves can be similar. And they can be powerful if we *give ourselves the opportunity to think* about them. How else do most personal wishes begin to come true?

SIGNPOST: *Relationships don't always help in ways we imagine they will*

Once we have connected with another in friendship, marriage, or a professional relationship, what do we do if we are not getting exactly what we think we want or need, especially in terms of support and companionship? If a relationship is not abusive, I suggest you stay in it. There are aspects of risk in all relationships. Though we can often predict what another will say or do, we can never be positively sure of another's response where our needs are concerned. Nor can we expect another to supply everything we need. Even our best relationships contain inequalities, imperfections, struggles, ebbs and flows, joys and sorrows. We can expect a lot from them, but must sometimes settle for less.

3. Find *your* pathway in faith.
Many people have found solace in suffering by connecting with the god of their beliefs. They talk about finding new strength and hope in practising an expression of faith. Convictions that God under-

stands and makes ultimate sense of all suffering, including mental illness, are often restful waters to be treasured and tapped.

A book I have found extremely helpful for people who would like to rekindle their religious faith but are having difficulty doing so, is *God of Surprises*, by Gerard W. Hughes (Darton, Longman & Todd 1985). This book gives solid suggestions for a spiritual journey that can complement your journey to recovery from your experience with mental illness.

SIGNPOST: Some religious counsel doesn't help

One cautionary note: sometimes pastoral workers and writers of religious books give inappropriate, even harmful, advice to those affected by mental illness. This advice includes messages such as, 'Just put yourself in the hands of God and you will be well' and 'If you had enough faith, you wouldn't be in this state' and 'Rid yourself of depression forever; learn to pray.' On more than one occasion, I have found myself having to counter the position that daily Bible reading, not medication, is what the person needs.

Underneath messages like these lies one or two assumptions: that those who pray and live 'faithfully' do not suffer mental illness; and that those whose lives weren't changed by prayer were not saying their prayers properly. This kind of thinking, in my opinion, lacks the benefit of basic knowledge about the dynamics of mental illness. Essentially, this kind of reasoning points to the person as being responsible for having a mental illness – in other words, the mental illness is attributed to the quality of the person's religious expression. This way of looking at a person struggling with mental illness can result in serious problems. For example, when a counsellor advises not taking medication such messages can bring havoc into the lives of patients and their families.

Let me be clear. I am not against messages suggesting that faith and prayer can help, but I am absolutely opposed to messages implying that individuals in some way bring about their mental illness because of their expression of faith.

My recommendation for those who are religiously inclined is, go ahead and be active in your faith but be sure to develop, if you haven't already, your critical powers when it comes to taking the advice of some religious counsellors.

We have now explored the first two stages of the grieving process; and have looked at ways and means of becoming aware of and working with denial and sadness. Now we will turn our attention to another grieving stage: anger.

FIVE

Be Angry!

Let's listen to the comments of three people as they talk about their anger and their experience with mental illness.

'You know, since we discussed anger in the group ... about how it's right to be angry about what's happened to me, I can see how much this makes sense. When I think about it, I see I've been very depressed about not feeling how I want to. I've been sick for so long. But angry? Well ... I'd get mad about not getting my way at home or here (in hospital), but I never really thought about being angry about being sick. Can you believe it? I never put being angry and being ill together! Now I know, because we talked about it, that I really have lots of anger about my illness.'

'My childhood was affected by my mother's psychiatric illness. I'm not blaming her; she did the best she could for us. But we could never bring anybody home after school because we never knew how she would be. When I was a teenager I kept thinking that if she got proper treatment, or if she would just try harder, she would behave normally. No one talked to me about her condition! Only now, and I'm thirty years old, have I finally found out the truth – that she has schizophrenia and that this is treatable but not curable. I feel very angry – about her having this devastating illness *and* about being kept in the dark about her condition.'

'Before, I never gave much of a passing thought to my life. Then I began to notice I was seeing things differently and doing things that were, I see now, really crazy. When things got bad enough I was brought to the hospital and I became a 'mental patient.' I felt degraded. Maybe it was the stigma. I know I was depressed about the whole ordeal. Now I'm thinking more about how my life has been disrupted, has been turned upside-down ... and how this happened to me! I never thought much about psychiatric problems before. Now I'm realizing that this is something not just to be angry about, but something to rage about! As far as expressing my anger, my rage, I'm trying to learn to do that, as you folks say, 'appropriately.' You know, at times I still 'act it out,' as my doctor puts it.'

Each of these speakers shows evidence of being well into the anger stage or phase of the conscious grieving process. They are focusing on specific points that relate directly to the mental illness experience in their lives. Having acknowledged these as causes for their anger, they are not telling themselves they shouldn't be angry. They have concluded that to be angry is clearly their justifiable right.

How did these people come to be comfortable with their anger? Like most of us, they had to learn that *being angry is okay*, and then, again like most of us, they had to look for ways to express and use their anger *constructively*.

SIGNPOST: We can learn how to handle anger

Before we enter the conscious grieving process about the experience of mental illness, it is extremely unusual to hear statements such as, 'I'm so angry that I have mental illness that I could _____,' or 'I'm angry because I didn't get the attention I needed from my parents. They had to focus more on my brother because he was mentally ill,' or 'I'm angry because I have a lot of educational goals and my illness prevents me from pursuing them.' It *is* usual, though, to hear people talk heatedly about wrong medications, helping professionals not caring (or being in it 'just for the money'), or one's family member simply being belligerent and stubborn. What is also common is their painfully high level of frustration.

Whenever I encounter people who are apparently experiencing a high degree of angst, I ask myself if they could be unconsciously on a 'grieving see-saw.' In other words, could they be moving between states of sadness and anger without attempting to resolve the basic issues underlying their emotions? Do they know anything about the normal grieving process? In most cases, when I have had the opportunity to put questions like these to people affected by mental illness, they confirm that they do feel they are on a see-saw. At this point it is helpful to explain both the dynamics and the benefits of the conscious grieving process.

From here we will review the necessary steps towards becoming rightfully and appropriately angry about the impact of mental illness in our lives. These steps begin, as they do in the case of denial and sadness, by looking at common ideas about anger that block its healthy, constructive expression. We will also look at guidelines that allow anger to take a welcome and proper place in our lives, as well as specific suggestions for using and expressing anger. Hopefully, you will also be able to find and affirm your own reasons for being angry. Though you may or may not find some clues in the examples given, I encourage you to *work actively* to discover what *your own* particular angering situations and issues are.

Before we arrive at the point of embracing and being comfortable with our anger, most of us need to rework our thinking about it. This is necessary because our culture so often bombards us with terribly underdeveloped and often harmful notions about these feelings.

A look at the different but equally problematic messages about anger given to women and men gives us a good idea about how and why we become handicapped in relation to anger. Females, both as children and as adults, are given a constant and clear message that anger is not an acceptable part of the picture of a desirable or ideal woman. This message (from parents, teachers, and clergy), spoken powerfully to women, says that no matter how legitimate their anger or how appropriate its expression, it should not be expressed or even *felt*.[1]

Garbled and unhealthy messages about anger are also routinely driven home to males. These messages range from the abhorrently violent (so often portrayed graphically on film) to the more subtly violent (war toys and other toy weapons). Admonitions such as, 'Big boys don't cry' (sometimes heard as 'Punch or be punched, but don't bawl if you hurt') have made men either duck their anger, completely avoid it, or express it in ways that are outright destructive.

In short, women are taught that anger, not just its expression, is wrong for them if they want to get on in life, while men get the message that destructive use of anger is generally what is expected of them – that is, as long as they are on the 'right side' of the fight.

When we consider the many unhelpful, misleading lessons we have learned about anger, we begin to see why we have such difficulty dealing with it. No wonder so many of us dislike ourselves or are afraid of ourselves when we feel anger welling up. No wonder we find ourselves saying, 'I'm sorry I got mad' instead of 'I was angry and I had a right to be angry.'

However, it is never too late. If we choose to, we can learn beneficial, constructive ways to express anger. I have known many people who have learned, through consciously grieving their experience with mental illness, that anger is as good and healthy an emotion as any. They have also learned that anger needs exercise. What follows are some tips to increase your 'anger fitness.'

SIGNPOST: You can use your anger positively

Consider these three basic principles about anger:

1. Anger has a legitimate place and function in our lives.

1 I believe that, even with the efforts of the women's movement to encourage women to express their anger and identify their issues (and maybe because some women have satisfactorily done this), women are still getting strongly conflicting messages about how to deal with their anger.

2. Anger is an unacceptable excuse for destructive behaviour.

3. Anger requires us to make choices about its use.

Grieving theorists have shown us evidence that feelings of anger about losses we have encountered form a stage or phase in the grieving process. They have observed that most people, having experienced denial and sadness about their losses, eventually feel angry about them. They describe how some people whose loved ones have died actually become angry at the dead relatives or friends for dying, and blame them for leaving them with their grief and loss. They can even find themselves mightily seething about the hole in their lives created by the death.

What lessons are we to learn from these observations about the place of anger in loss? There are at least two:

1. Whatever form our loss takes, our anger is normal and healthy.

2. When we are consciously grieving our experience with mental illness, making use of our anger is an unavoidable part of the journey to recovery.

SIGNPOST: Deal with anger step by step

When it comes to using anger efficiently – that is, to use it to move ourselves towards our goal of recovery – we must learn to take it a step at a time. Here are those essential steps:

1. Name and claim your angry feelings.
You are feeling angry for a reason. Because of mental illness you have had to leave your job, your career has been put on hold, your income has been reduced, you have shelled out a lot of money for an ill relative in order to cover unexpected expenses, friends and relatives don't treat you the way they used to, you hate what your illness is doing to you. The list, short or long, contains realities that have meant crushing hardship.

Remember, like the conscious processing of any grieving feeling, anger deserves to be dealt with thoroughly and respectfully. Also keep in mind that recognizing anger can be difficult. For one thing, the anger may be and often is one of a number of feelings experienced at the same time. Disappointment, guilt, sadness, and fear are often anger's travelling companions. Nevertheless, once a person says, 'I am angry,' then he or she can begin to sort through and examine the cause(s) of the anger.

2. Look for the cause of your anger.
Looking for what's underlying the feelings of anger can have many benefits, including some *unexpected* and *welcome ones.*

Sally, a person who had suffered a chronic mental illness for some years, found that making a list of the consequences of her illness helped her name and claim her anger. She detailed how the illness had affected her personally: She had lost her steady, well-paying job; she had had to change her residence; and she had lost friends, including her boyfriend. Her list also included the imperfect treatments she endured and the inadequate resources available in her geographic area. Making this list left Sally with no doubts that she had plenty to be angry about.

What happened when Sally realized her anger was absolutely appropriate? She not only made gains through sharpening her insight about the consequences of her mental illness, she also worked to put her anger to use. As she put it, instead of 'blaming everyone and everything' for her circumstances, she decided to take some control of the efforts to improve them. She also did a lot of work learning ways of recognizing and curtailing her tendency to paranoid thinking.

Sally's positive experience illustrates how conscious effort to work with anger can help to heighten insight. Not only does it help us understand better what has happened to our lives, it also steers us in new, constructive directions, enabling us to manage our lives in more satisfying ways. Energized and actually *empowered by anger,* the person suffering a mental illness first hand can also decide to develop his or her existing insight further.

3. See in anger its signal for decision-making.
Key to learning how to employ anger constructively is to recognize its presence as early as possible – that is, to recognize its early 'sparks' or 'surges' and to see this as a signal to start making decisions. Recognizing anger can be the start of a fact-finding mission to determine how others have handled news about their psychiatric diagnoses, to learn about prospects for rehabilitation and the availability of other resources in your community, and to find out what you can realistically expect. This will happen, however, only if you have *decided to use anger in these ways.*

4. Find a safe place!
When patients and their caregivers attempt to put the energy of their anger to useful purpose, they may find they are fuelling their anger. At the risk of sounding like an old broken record, I must point out that this experience, like most experiences in grieving, is *normal.* The exercise of making a list of underlying causes for our anger *naturally* has the effect of raising our 'anger temperature.' This is why, in order to use anger consciously *and* constructively, we need to find a safe place – a place to give ourselves a chance to simmer down, sort out our issues, rank them, and then make choices. Safe places may be found in bathrooms, bedrooms, kitchens, studies, streets, parks – any place that provides a calm, supportive atmosphere. Consider inviting someone you trust to be with you. This not only makes a safe place more safe, but also can be of real value in helping you make *constructive* decisions.

5. Choose a constructive route for your anger.
Though the focus of this chapter is the *constructive use* of anger, this does not mean that I believe we should ignore the unconstructive or frankly destructive sentiments that we all experience from time to time. On the contrary, let's look at those times when we decide to take a negative course, such as hurting someone back (getting even), giving up on the recovery process (copping out of a rehabilitation program), or holding another person responsible for our psychiatric experience (blaming mother).

In my work with patients and their families, if I sense that someone is about to use anger unconstructively, I recommend as strongly
as possible that a thorough and careful look be taken before pro-
ceeding. Ninety-nine times out of a hundred, when people examine
their intentions closely, they discover that they don't simply want to
get even, to give up, or to blame. Rather, they want to get the anger-
causing situation *successfully* over with.[2]

Let's look at an excellent example of moving away from destructive anger and towards beginning the search for options to solve a
problem once and for all.

Ken appeared at my office door, obviously upset and talking
about wanting to 'deck' his apartment manager. He had been working on avoiding 'acting out' his anger – that is, expressing anger in
ways that got him into trouble with people. On this occasion, he
made it clear that he wanted to use my office as a safe place. He
also wondered aloud if I could stay with him to help him handle his
feelings.

By giving himself permission to take time out 'away from the
scene,' and inviting my supportive counsel, Ken had given himself a
chance to discover that the last thing he wanted was more problems. Once he had simmered down, he needed only to think of the
web of trouble he would be in if he assaulted his apartment manager to change his plan of action. Ken thought about the probabil-
ity of an assault charge and the possibility of conviction and a
criminal record. He also considered the fact that abusing someone
physically or emotionally never solves anything. Ken began to focus
on how he could make constructive use of his anger.

6. Plot out a concrete plan for using your anger.
Once a person makes a decision to take a constructive route in
expressing anger, further decisions need be made. When we ask in
group work for examples of successful and satisfying expressions of
anger, 'taking a walk' and 'punching a punching bag' are nearly

2 If, after reading this chapter, you still want to get even, give up, or blame, please seek professional help for this problem. As long as you retain reactions such as 'I don't care' or 'I
just want to give the so-and-so a taste of his own medicine!' you are clearly in danger of
harming yourself and others.

always mentioned. These are excellent starting points, but they are just that: starting points. Use them, but don't stop there. Taking walks and punching pillows or bags are wonderful exercises when our anger reaches the boiling-point. However, they will not resolve long-term or lasting problems. So, you say, what does? Here's another signpost.

SIGNPOST: *When we use anger constructively, one decision leads to another*

After you have reduced the heat of your anger, try this exercise to help put it to use.

EXERCISE 8:

The next time you are on that walk, jabbing at the punching bag, or are in the safe place you have found to deal with your anger, ask the two key coping questions:

• How can I help myself cope with _____?

• Are there ways I can use this experience of anger constructively?

Fill in the end of the first question with your own angry feeling (frustration, rage, bitterness, revenge), as well as the details of the situation that is causing you to feel angry. Remind yourself that there is nothing wrong with your anger. Then ask yourself if you want or need to be in a continuous rage or even in a simmering state of wrath. If you give yourself this time for reflection, satisfactory answers are likely to come to you, along with suggestions for relieving the intensity of your angry feelings.

Your answers to the second question will help you put your anger to practical, constructive use. For this reason, the more *specific detail* you can come up with, the better. Remember to keep your solutions *realizable* – that is, they must be achievable considering your day-to-day life and taking into account things such as your finances, energy, and responsibilities.

When you are focusing on your anger and are serious about

using it in a constructive way, you will find that you won't stop until you have figured out ways to bring some peace to yourself, and perhaps to others. The simmering-down effect that comes with taking the first step on your 'exercising it off' walk will bring you in closer touch with your ability to sort out constructive plans from unconstructive ones. This is basic *anger management* practice – in other words, it is helpful in any situation that makes us angry. Remember, when we are consciously grieving the experience of mental illness, we must ask ourselves this question: How can I use my anger constructively?

Ultimately, we must each find our individual answers to this question. However, there are several strategies that have brought relief to many thousands of people, *and* have helped them use their anger in a positive way. Let's look at them.

SIGNPOST: Anger has energy you can use

1. Join a support and information group.
What do groups do for those of us who have experienced mental illness?

• They provide an opportunity to learn how others have coped with issues similar to our own. We find out we are not the only ones with problems dealing with mental illness.

• They give us a place, not only where we can vent our frustrations and other reactions, but also where we can receive assurances that our reactions are normal. Many find this particularly valuable after finding themselves misunderstood for so long.

• They provide a forum for the exchange of vital information about the nature of mental illnesses and the availability of treatments, formal psychiatric rehabilitation programs, and other resources.

As a social worker, I well know that many people think at first that groups are not for them. I also know very well that many who were once strongly resistant to attending groups have eventually found that support and information groups have become their lifeline. In them, their educational needs are served and friendships are formed – a welcome surprise to those who have become isolated or ostracized. As discussed earlier, we can't get away from the fact that we are *social beings*. Because we are social beings, we not only *have social needs*, we also *deserve* and *require* that these needs be met.

Many kinds of groups have formed around various issues with respect to mental illness. These include information groups, support groups, advocacy groups, and 'survivor' groups. Some are the self-help type, while others are professionally led. An increasing number of 'coping with mental illness' groups are facilitated through partnerships composed of people affected first hand by the illness and professional helpers.

At different points in your recovery journey you will have different needs. It may be to your advantage to move on from one group to another *or* to take a rest from group involvement. Of course, no one group can be *the* answer to *all* your stresses. Expect, though, to find some support in meeting and coming to know others whose experience is similar to yours.

Be sure to *make use of educational groups by doing them your way.* I have always found it helpful to try and find at least one useful or interesting point in a speaker's address, or to manufacture my own using the speaker's comments as reference points. Looking for one gem of wisdom will keep me tuned in on occasions when speakers are not to my taste or when I disagree with most of what is being said. Additionally, I have found that times like these are opportunities to review and perhaps change my thinking.

Keep in mind that though some information might be old hat to you, information framed in a new way may still contain important items for your journey to recovery. It may be helpful also to look at 'heard it before' information as a mini refresher course. And if someone is talking, for example, about a way of doing things that you have already learned *and* faithfully practised, it is a good time to give yourself a big, affirming pat on the back!

2. Seek out a professional counsellor who has the time, patience,

and knowledge to help you work through the anger stage of your grieving.

You will recognize this person. He or she is the one who approves of your anger and is willing to help direct you to use your anger's energy towards constructive, desirable goals. On the other hand, if a would-be helper confronts you about your 'inappropriate' expression of anger and does not help you explore ways to use it constructively, or does not help you rehearse your way through the action you have chosen to take, I would suggest you move on to another counsellor. Remember, before doing so, to take your courage in hand and tell your present counsellor why you are moving on.

3. Write a journal.

Journals are great places for reaching for your feelings, describing them, labelling them, and figuring out how they connect to your losses. Many people who have suffered physical (including sexual) abuse sometimes use journalling to write letters to those who have offended them. They find that writing letters to the offender is a path to healing. These letters, often never sent, can be useful receptacles for innermost feelings of hurt, outrage, confusion, abandonment, betrayal, and loss of innocence.

Journal entries can be as long or short as you want them to be. You can write as much or as little detail as you care to. Take care not to criticize your writing style or the content of your entries. This endeavour is your private affair, not an exam! Do give some thought to how you can keep your journal safe from the eyes of others. It is also a good idea to date each entry. This will enable you to see and better appreciate your struggles and progress.

4. Never stop educating yourself!

Keep learning about the particular mental illness that has affected your life. Make enquiries about the latest research findings. Find out about its dynamics. Learn how others worked their way through to recovery, survival, and wholeness. Keep in mind that while no one else's way can be yours exactly, picking up even a hint or two from others can be like having that very valuable loose change just when you need it.

The shelves of public libraries often have a good supply of literature about dealing with mental illness. I recommend heartily that you find what is available in your area. But just one important note of caution: If you find the subject matter disagreeable, put it back on the library shelf. Unfortunately, some self-help material is written in a blaming, confrontational style that won't help you.

5. Investigate your community resources and find out what's happening.
Find out what your community is doing about mental illness. More and more often, treatment centres are relying on information from those directly affected by mental illness, in order to help improve their services – an outreach that is long overdue.

6. Consider bridge building.
In most communities, growing pains are felt when various sectors working with mental illness attempt to exchange information and carry out action plans. For example, consumers of psychiatric services may focus on faults in existing services without suggesting realistic alternatives. As well, basic disagreements about treatments can sometimes pose a serious threat to health (advice to go off medication). What is particularly troubling is that sometimes there seems to be no middle ground. Professional caregivers who rarely make themselves available for an exchange of information contribute to this problem.

Professional helpers, and other caregivers too, have often separated themselves from people who suffer psychiatric illness first hand. Undoubtedly, there are a number of reasons for this. I sometimes think we separate ourselves because as caregivers we do not give much thought to the possibility of being affected in our personal lives by psychiatric illness. In other words, we unconsciously assume that mental illness only happens to others.

Those who have the experience of mental illness to deal with and are not professionals sometimes just say nothing. In many cases they have given up trying to explain themselves or to get the help they need.

It is time we looked at doing some bridge building. It is time that patients and caregivers (family, friends, and professionals) used the energy of their anger to connect in meaningful, constructive ways. Lip-service and bad-mouthing must be set aside. They don't work! On the other hand, authentic, wholehearted dialogue *can* produce results and it must be initiated in all sectors dealing with mental illness if we want to make a constructive difference.

Up to this point we have looked at and had a chance to practise conscious uses of our grieving in its denial, sadness, and anger phases. Before we go on to the resolution or acceptance phase, let's consider the problem of fear.

SIX

Taming Fear

Fear's threads weave themselves throughout the grieving process as it relates to mental illness. These are strong threads that are occasionally clearly noticeable and recognizable, but are more often masked by denial, sadness, and anger. Fear, unrecognized and unresolved, can have us going nowhere on our recovery journey, or going off in many directions on routes that, with hindsight, we would rather not have travelled.

Over and over again, I hear people talking about theirs fears as they relate to their experiences with mental illness:

'I'm afraid the doctors won't get the medications right for my daughter.'

'I'm afraid to take on my illness.' (A patient's reason not to enter a psychiatric rehabilitation program.)

'We can't leave her alone for fear of what will happen while we're away.' (A parent's fear for a child who attempted suicide.)

'I'm scared that my brother will end up on the streets.'

'I'm paralysed with fear that I'll have a full-fledged episode of mental illness again.'

In many ways, and for several years, fear directed the course of my life. I was afraid that if I started to make any changes – getting a paying job, going back to school, doing volunteer work – that I would become so enthusiastic, so overwhelmed, so serious, so depressed, or 'so something' that I would trip myself into another episode of acute illness. Thus, my way of living was to remain safe and stuck. This might have been what I needed to do for a while, but surely not for ten years! What I did need to do was learn to deal with my fear. Until I did so, my efforts to work from and with the healthy parts of myself (including my fear) and to take risks were handicapped.

This chapter looks at ways to deal with your fears in ways that are purposeful and useful. We will be looking at some common grounds for fear in the experience of mental illness, and we will come to see that these are, in most cases, *reasonable*. We will also explore the problem of stigma, to better understand what it is and what we can do about it.

SIGNPOST: Our grounds for fear are usually reasonable

The fears of those who suffer mental illness cover a variety of issues, including fear of:

- never recovering

- never recovering enough to fulfil one's dreams

- becoming mentally ill again upon reaching recovery

- damage to reputation

- damage to relationships

- thinking the worst-case prognosis applies to oneself

- life now being always unpredictable

- the illness being obvious to everyone

This list touches only the surface. As a friend pointed out, any list of fears related to mental illness should also include fear of more specific things, fear of leaving home (as in the case of phobias and obsessive-compulsive behaviours), and, in her case, the paralysing fear of not being able to sleep. Indeed, our fears can range from being afraid 'no one will sit with me in the cafeteria' (so we eat by ourselves day after day, depriving ourselves of the companionship we need) to avoiding anything new in case it leads to another episode of illness.

Those who are affected secondarily by mental illness – family, friends, and even some professional caregivers – often express fears and doubts about what the future holds for them. Initially relieved to hear the diagnosis of a loved one's psychiatric condition, caregivers often find fear replacing the relief.

The presence of fear often comes to light in family-information group sessions. The mother of a young man in hospital for the first time approached me after one of these sessions. Tearful and anxious, she said, 'I just can't believe that my son will not get over this breakdown. The doctor said it might be schizophrenia. What I'm learning here makes me so afraid for him ... for his future and mine.'

This woman certainly had grounds for fear. She had learned that evening that her son's illness might well be *chronic*, and that though efforts to find a cure for schizophrenia are underway (in spite of very limited funding), treatments are not perfect. All I could do that evening for this distressed mother was offer a few words of support and remain with her for awhile.

The fears of many family members take on a special burden because they are connected to the family's anticipation that their loved ones will do something harmful either to themselves or others. In some cases, unfortunate previous experiences with harmful behaviour (for example, suicidal threats and/or attempts) profoundly compound the fear experience.

SIGNPOST: Learn to let fear be the fuel, not the driver

For everyone affected by mental illness, it is important to come to *own* and *wrestle with* fear so that two things happen:

1. It is not *the* driving force of your life.

2. Whatever is at the bottom of your fear can be used to plan how you are going to handle your fearful situation.

When people talk about being afraid, it is not unusual to find that they have difficulty identifying the specifics of the fear. When I ask both patients and family members what their particular fears are about, their answers are sometimes in the form of hesitant guesses about what might happen. At other times, they have no answers at all. When my questions are avoided, I wonder if the person is so deeply afraid of the possible outcome of the illness (suicide or some other form of harm to oneself or to others) that *even talking about these fears* may seem too threatening.

Whatever our reasons for not being readily able or willing to grapple with the sources of our fears, we need to remember that fear, if not confronted, can and often does seriously hamper our efforts to recover.

The next two exercises are designed to help you put *whatever it is you are fearing into clear focus* and to assist you to develop ways of coping with your fears and using them to recover.

EXERCISE 9:

If possible, do this exercise in the company of someone you trust. As you work through it, don't get discouraged if the results that come to mind seem too inconsequential to be considered objects of fear. Many of us suffer from a build-up of small fears, which can have the same paralysing impact as one major fear (such as doing physical harm to yourself or others). Remember that, bit by bit and step by step, your fears can be tamed – that is, handled – when you have rendered them into manageable chunks. It may be helpful to think of yourself as a carver, whittling away *gradually* at your feelings of fear; imagine that you are beginning to take charge of your fears, and not the other way around.

1. Start the exercise by getting into your safe place.

2. Bring yourself to a calm state by breathing deliberately and

slowly. Try as much as possible to empty your mind of all thoughts that are not related to your fear.

3. After a few minutes, when you feel relaxed, *focus* on identifying only *one* subject of your *fear*. Do not allow unhelpful thoughts to take over (for example, ones that tell you this is a useless exercise). When they do, consider them only mildly bothersome distractions and return to focusing. Continue until the image of one subject of fear comes to the forefront of your mental landscape.

Repeat these steps as often as necessary, until one subject of fear is clear. Once it comes into focus, you are back in the driver's seat and in position to ask *the key coping question*: 'How can I help myself cope with my fear of _____?'

Asking the key question in the face of one particular fear will lead you to the point where you can begin building the coping skills you need to deal with your fearful situation. In other words, it puts you in a position of power. Now, *you* are deciding what *you can do* with your fear. Repeat this exercise every time you become aware of a new fear or traces of one previously dealt with. Remember, dealing with fear requires a continual, conscious, 'whittling' activity.

The next exercise is designed to help you test each clearly focused fear, particularly if you are feeling that it is in some way silly, groundless, or unreasonable.

EXERCISE 10:

1. Stare what you are afraid of 'in the face.'

2. Ask, 'Is this really something to be fearful of?'

3. If your answer is no, picture yourself putting what was frightening you into an imaginary garbage can. Do this every time this fear, or a trace of it, returns.

4. If your answer is yes, welcome the fear as the bearer of an important message. Our fears can be among our greatest teachers as we journey to recovery. Explore the fear. Find out what it has to tell

you. Look for ways to unlock the trap that that particular fear has held you in. If no solutions become apparent, reach out for help.

Help can be a phone call away, particularly if you seek the services of a self-help organization. (Try your local chapter of the Schizophrenia Society of Canada, the Association for Relatives and Friends of the Emotionally and Mentally Ill (ARFEMI) in Australia, the National Alliance for the Mentally Ill in the United States, the National Schizophrenia Fellowship (SANE) in Great Britain.) Many individuals and families have found not only some answers to their initial questions but also a virtual means of survival through the networks these organizations offer.

SIGNPOST: Give serious consideration to safety issues

If you as a caregiver find that your fear has its grounds in issues related to safety (for example, if you fear that you or somebody else may be hurt by the one who is ill or that he or she will commit suicide), do not ignore these fears. Advise professional staff at the patient's treatment facility, or, if this is not possible (for example, if you aren't familiar with a treatment centre, or your loved one has never been treated), find out from a nearby mental health agency or your own physician what legal routes you can take to have your ill family member examined, and follow one of them. Take advantage of professional advice regarding all your safety concerns. Your own safety and that of your loved one are paramount!

If the person who has mental illness is living with you and you are afraid for reasons of safety, it is important that you seek ways of making the situation safe. This may mean a move to supportive housing for your loved one. Having worked with many families through this kind of transition, I know it can have many repercussions: guilt, shame, sorrow – even more fears. Still, these feelings *can be dealt with*. Certainly, all of them pale in comparison to the potentially tragic outcomes which signalled the need for change in the first place.

Social workers in most hospitals and helping agencies have mandates that deal with the concerns of family members and keep them abreast of the ways and means of putting families in touch with community service resources. At my workplace we recommend that the social workers on a treatment team be contacted, rather than the psychiatrist, because they (and not psychiatrists) are the professionals who have had extensive training to service family needs. Of course, not all social workers know the dynamics of mental illness and its social dimensions, but those who work in psychiatric settings know that family members need and deserve information about mental health laws, community resources for housing and financial assistance, and ways to access these and other support services. Some also have expertise acting as mediators to help resolve problems among family members that arise because mental illness is present in the family.

But, a word of caution: be sure the professional helpers you choose do not use therapy methods that essentially blame someone (often the mother) for being over-protective, over-involved, or inadequate. Though family problems such as dysfunctional parenting can be related to some forms of mental illness, research has shown that in the overwhelming majority of cases, it does not cause major mental illness. If you are concerned about what is being recommended to you, get a second opinion. And please do not accept any blame. In all likelihood, you have been doing the best you can in very difficult circumstances.

SIGNPOST: Tame a fear by naming it

With hindsight, I can see that my own experience with fear was a problem for two reasons: either I could not find the right words to talk about my fears; or I had vague notions that if I did talk about them, I would receive responses that minimized my concerns (for example, 'Don't think about that now,' or 'Don't be silly,' or 'It won't happen.').

My fears *and their resolutions* provided particularly enlightening lessons to me personally, but most took me by surprise because they came by accident. I hope that by recounting some parts of this leg of my journey, your lessons will be learned less accidentally than mine.

My greatest fear after major episodes of mental illness, as mentioned before, was becoming ill again. Only when I finally brought this fear out into the clear light of day, *named it, and claimed it*, did resolution of that fear begin.

It happened in our home one evening after dinner. My husband and I were once again talking about my future. Returning to school became the subject. As usual I was very hesitant and full of 'I wish I could' sentiments: 'I might get sick again. Course material might send me into mania. I might fail and then get depressed, and I don't ever want to go through that again.' For one reason or another I blurted out what I had not been willing or able to say before: 'I'm afraid I'll get sick again if I go back to school.'

To the casual observer this would hardly seem significant, but it was critical to the resolution of my fear, as was my husband's reply. Supportive as always, he put his thoughts in the form of questions: 'How do you know that your chances of getting sick again will occur at regular intervals? Maybe your illness will never happen again, or maybe it will – according to a timetable of the number of years between your bouts squared?' I remembered enough math that this statistic gave me some hope. I began challenging my fear by asking myself questions such as, 'What if I were to get sick again, not within four years (the interval between my severest episodes) but in four times four years?' Somehow I was reassured by the thought of a sixteen-year interval between attacks of mental illness. I can't now explain exactly why that little mathematical formulation gave my previously paralysing fear enough pause so that I could begin to make some plans.

Later, it was my husband's 'How do you know ...?' question that continued to sustain me. In fact, I still use it to calm myself to this day. Thinking about what I did know about the future (which was *exactly nothing* for sure) had prompted me to think more about taking risks in planning my future. Gradually, too, my thinking about getting sick again began to focus on what I could do to avoid acute illness, if this were in fact within my capacity.

Here, I want to emphasize what I believe is a very important point about personal responsibility in managing one's own illness. Some authors of self-help books believe that each of us is responsible for our illnesses. I strongly disagree. I believe that most mental illnesses have a life of their own, that they surface in spite of state-of-the-art care *and* the efforts by patients to keep their illnesses at bay. In my opinion, people who suffer depression are among those who are often misunderstood, and sometimes outrightly blamed by caregivers who use a 'You've chosen to be depressed' line of therapy. I do believe that most all of us can learn to do something to help ourselves in the face of mental illness. I do not believe people choose to be mentally ill.

SIGNPOST: Lessons about dealing with fear

What important messages did I harvest from dealing with my fear? There were several. One that is now obvious (but wasn't at the time): to fear another episode of acute illness is reasonable. I also learned that to feel afraid is more than okay – it is a survival instinct. I needed it to make plans that work for me. Fear taught me to believe in my own advice to myself, such as: take what care I can not to become ill again. I learned to disregard false reassurances, such as, 'It won't happen again.' Over time, other lessons that have evolved from facing my fears have been equally as character building as the first one I learned that evening with the help of my husband. Here's a summary.

1. In naming and claiming our fears, we take responsibility for our feelings of fear and can then tame them so that they are not running our lives.

2. In order to tame fears to manageable shape and proportion, we will, on some occasions, need to open ourselves to the support of others.

3. Often, we can take measures to make acute episodes of mental illness a remote possibility rather than an inevitability.

4. We can open up, not only to conventional psychiatric help, but also to other kinds of help, such as rehabilitation coaching, self-help books, and inspirational audio and visual tapes.

5. We can look at the ways we have successfully managed fear in the past and know that we have reason to believe we can handle current fears.

6. If we profess a belief in God, we can seek help from God when, for example, we are suddenly feeling frightened and alone. Recall-

ing, at times like this, that we are not alone and that we don't have to handle everything ourselves, can lighten the burden of fear.

SIGNPOST: Dealing with stigma

Stigma, often captured in questions such as, 'What if my/her/his mental-patient status becomes public knowledge?' stems from fear *based on ignorance* about mental illness and treatment for mental illness. In other words, stigma about mental illness does not stand on reasonable (including humanitarian) grounds.

Ignorance about mental illness is rampant. Before ever personally encountering it, most of us hardly give it a thought. Why is this? I am not sure there is any one clear answer. Sometimes the questions asked about stigma lead only to more questions. Looking at how news of mental illness is handled sometimes helps to sharpen some of our notions as to the why's and wherefore's of stigma. When someone in the neighbourhood has a 'breakdown,' it is usually kept hush-hush for one reason or another. Few, if any, become wiser because of this experience. From time to time our whole society is warned that revealing episodes of mental illness can have extremely dire consequences. A case in point: American vice-presidential hopeful Tom Eagleton, who was forced out of the running because he had sought psychiatric treatment for depression.

Examples such as Tom Eagleton's experience make us think again before disclosing any psychiatric history that 'lurks' in our individual histories. While some of us may be pretty well assured that we won't be kicked out as Tom Eagleton was, most of us have a sense that at the very least our credibility will be put into question. So most of us keep quiet.[1]

What can we do with stigma? Realistically, can we make it go away? Probably not. But, perhaps some of us, like Mayor Cain, can begin to put a big dent into it by educating others. Some of us begin

---

1 A wonderful exception was contained in the words of Claudette Cain upon her election as mayor of Gloucester, Ontario. As reported by the *Ottawa Citizen* (18 November 1991): 'Cain says she emerged from the experience [of mental illness] "better than new." But she watches out for symptoms of depression – in herself and in others ... "I feel that I'm a better person for having gone through it."'

this process by sharing details of our experience only with trusted friends.

This sharing often (though not always) has positive results. Many report that stigma doesn't exist among friends as much as they believed it would. People with mental illness tell stories time and again about how they were pleasantly surprised and relieved by the support they received when they shared their experience. For the most part, this was what happened to me. In fact, as I gradually came to talk more openly about my psychiatric history, I found myself encouraged, in the true sense of that word. The stories some of my friends told me – stories about their own or another's experience with the world of psychiatric illness – let me know that others had learned to handle the experience, had gotten through it (or were still attempting to get through it), and had even come to enjoy some sense of achievement again. In all my experience through recovery, nothing has been more empowering than the example of others who have travelled and continue to travel the recovery journey.

SIGNPOST: *Some people won't understand*

Like most people who suffer mental illness, I have not been spared exposure to some who do not understand. While I have never felt totally shunned by anyone, I have received unhelpful messages from some people who presume to know about possible causes of my illness. For example, 'You are a very intense person. Should you be working in a high-stress field?' and 'You've always taken on loads of responsibility, maybe too much.'

In spite of my best explanations and protests that my illness had more to do with body chemistry than what I did or how much, some people simply failed to understand that my experience was not my fault, my husband's fault, or my parents' fault for raising me the way they did. Nor was it related to my workplace. Others have attempted to protect me from possible consequences should others find out the 'horrid truth' about my past. One professional colleague even advised me not to tell an administrator about my history, even though we worked in a place where respect for people with mental illness should have been abundant. I had found stigma in a most unexpected place! After I thought about what my colleague had said, I decided to let her advice serve as a reminder that:

1. I have the right to be selective about just who I care to tell my story to.

2. Being selective can be wise, given that *stigma does exist, even in the least expected places.*

SIGNPOST: We can choose to go public

Moving beyond our trusted friends and acquaintances in an attempt to challenge the stigma of mental illness is a worthy task. However, if we do participate in this way, let's make it as easy on ourselves as possible, beginning perhaps with acknowledging that we are never going to 'change the whole world.'

A way that helps many of us when we do something to make our world a better place is to do it with others. As mentioned in the last chapter, there is now a growing psychiatric survivor/consumer movement. People who have been affected by mental illness are now getting together to deal with some of their vital concerns: the availability of appropriate supportive housing, homelessness, job opportunities, modes of treatment, treatment availability, and poverty. In many communities, groups can be found that are both advocating for better services and attempting to educate the public about mental illness concerns. Joining the work of such a group, if you feel ready, can give you the chance to make a meaningful contribution to public education with respect to mental illness.

If you do decide to tackle the stigma of mental illness, consider these guidelines:

1. It is your right to be selective about who you talk to about your experience with mental illness.

2. If you choose to educate the public, either join a group or organize one.

3. In a group situation, if you feel you cannot or do not want to participate in certain group efforts, don't let yourself be pushed or pulled to do so. Give yourself permission to 'sit out' any activity you are not comfortable with. Remember, when it comes to your life, you want to be in the driver's seat.

The next chapter takes us over the last leg of the recovery journey: acceptance.

SEVEN

Acceptance: The Journey Continues

'I can never accept this illness!' (The statement of a person suffering a chronic mental illness.)

'Patients should *never* accept their illness. If they do, they will just give up.' (One mental health practitioner's belief.)

'She seems to have accepted the label of her illness, but she has no motivation or goals. Wouldn't she be more inclined to get a job if she hadn't reconciled to her illness? We think her health would improve if she would go back to her job.' (Comment by a parent.)

Over the last few years, as I have attempted to teach people whose lives are touched in different ways by the mental illness experience, I have heard statements like these many, many times. Now, when I'm talking to individuals or groups about the conscious grieving process, I look forward to questions and statements like these because I see them as opportunities to clarify what acceptance means in the mental illness context.

SIGNPOST: Being clear about what acceptance means

Let's first understand that acceptance does not mean giving unqualified approval about the presence of mental illness in our lives. In the stage of acceptance, we are not saying we are glad about the experience. Granted, a few can say in retrospect that their misfortune was a blessing in disguise, as Mayor Cain did. But is it realistic to think we are all able or willing to speak approvingly of the personal experience mental illness has brought us? I don't think so. In my opinion, each of us may develop some sense of approval within ourselves about the experience – for example, as we make efforts to learn to cope in healthy ways with mental illness's consequences, ways we would not have bothered with unless the illness had occurred. But to get to the point of saying, 'I'm glad it happened' may be, at least for many of us, impossible.

What is the meaning of acceptance, then, in the context of this conscious grieving process? It means facing the realities brought about by the presence of mental illness, and then building and practising coping skills so that recovery can be achieved and maintained.

It is also important, at this point, to think again about the meaning of recovery. As discussed in the Introduction, each of us needs to develop his or her own definition of recovery – because recovery is *unique* to each individual. We know that recovering from the impact or trauma of mental illness is not the same as recovering from the mental illness itself. By consciously grieving our individual mental illness experiences, we are seeking ways to bring a sense of restoration to our lives. We are aiming to heal the wounds this experience has brought to our sense of our selves, or, if you prefer, to our spirits or souls. We are giving ourselves permission to get in touch with our feelings of grief in order to regain a sense of control in our lives. This is recovery. We have recovered, or perhaps *discovered*, a new and precious *sense of ourselves*. And this sense, often beginning as a fragile sense of a still-fragile self, puts us in position to cope with and manage our experience with mental illness – whether we suffer it ourselves or care for someone who does. This, too, means recovery.

To my mind, recovery and the acceptance phase of grieving are similar and cannot exist without one another. Both are stages *in process* that require continued conscious effort if they are to remain with us. Both are best tested for their presence in our lives by our taking into account not only our achievements (small and large) but also the *efforts* we make to achieve them.

SIGNPOST: Insight, activity, and affirmation yield acceptance

We are now going to take a closer look at acceptance by exploring its major elements – insight, activity, and affirmation – taking each in turn.

SIGNPOST: Sustain recovery through insight

Awareness and understanding of the realities brought about through the experience of mental illness, commonly called 'insight,' form the foundation of acceptance. These realities include those losses related to mental illness as well as the loss that mental illness is in itself. Personal abilities, dreams, expectations, savings, status, friendships, jobs, family, and residence are among the targets for the fallout of mental illness. Realizing and processing these tough realities – that is, coming to know how our own experience with mental illness has affected us and others around us, and what needs to be done to cope – is what having insight means.

It is important here to review briefly a few of the points about denial – lack of insight – that we covered earlier. Remember, what can become unhealthy for any individual affected by the experience of mental illness – and I emphasize that this applies to caregivers and patients – is a *prolonged* stay in any of the early stages of grieving, including denial. As well, a *lack of insight*, often simply called denial, is a *normal* part of this grieving process. It is also, as psychiatrists explain, a part of the normal make-up of some mental illnesses. It is of utmost importance to keep in mind that grieving, including denying loss, is what each of us *needs to do to survive our losses for as long as it takes* each of us to do so.

The moral of this last point: Let us be very careful and very gentle when we make judgments about someone's (or our own) length of stay in any grieving stage, including denial.

Insight about the mental illness experience can come suddenly or gradually. Sometimes it is the way a particular problem is worded by a certain person that quickly leads us to a new and more wholesome picture of what has been and is happening. Just remember that insight development can take years.

Here is how one person with mental illness described how he gained insight:

> It took me so long to understand what had happened to bring me into hospital ... I had rejected all that my family was trying to say. I thought all of them, including my parents, were making things up because they all seemed to have been giving me such a hassle at home. I changed these ideas about my family.
>
> I still think that some of what you call my paranoia had some basis in fact. But I do understand that to be healthy I must try to listen to what others I once trusted are saying. Actually, I still don't believe everything, but I do listen and I do try to trust them.

My own insight development included both the sudden arrivals and the gradual (usually *very* gradual) dawnings of insight. I remember agreeing swiftly and unexpectedly with one of my nurses, that to believe someone was trying to shoot me didn't make sense. Up to that point, as I said earlier, I was convinced that my view of the world was right: a hired gun was in just the right place for the kill. Why that nurse's words, at that moment, helped me get past that piece of delusional thinking is still a mystery to me. Nor can I account for other sudden insights and experiences, other than to say that I understood the way a view different from my own was put to me, and perhaps was open enough to hear it at those moments. (Yes, the medication was probably doing some work, too.) But for the most part, the development of my insight has come about gradually *and* with a lot of consciously deliberate exploration.

Once seeds of insight are planted, we can nurture them. I believe we *must* nurture insight through reflection, study, and discussion, at least occasionally, in order to sustain recovery.

How do we keep our insights related to mental illness in working order? For those of us who suffer mental illness first hand, I recommend beginning with a very useful, though somewhat painful, practice: making an effort to recall the beginnings of the episodes of illness. This practice helps us discover and know our own individual early signs of illness: for example, tendencies to isolate ourselves, to believe nobody understands, to become more excited than usual, to be unusually more emotional (tearful, angry, *overly* joyful), to eat or sleep more or less than usual, to experience changes in our sexual habits, or to spend excessive amounts of money or none at all. Reminding ourselves of early signs of previous episodes of illness can serve to help us recognize that we need help *now*, when there is a good possibility that an oncoming acute episode of illness can be prevented.

A priest was the first to suggest that I practise attempting to recall the circumstances present (both within and around me) at the beginning of my bouts of illness. At the same time he told me that he also had psychological problems, and that doing this had helped him. (I will always be grateful to him for sharing these things with me.) At the time, I protested that I had become sick so fast I didn't know what had happened. He encouraged me to try anyway. I didn't at first, and it was a long time before I did. It still hurts to go over moments I would rather forget. But I am certain I would not have come to know myself, including the early warning signs of my psychiatric disability, if I hadn't deliberately attempted to recall those moments. I found that I *could* find valuable pieces among my memory's store about 'what happened.' These have led me to ways of being, thinking, and doing which in turn have helped me keep my psychiatric disability in check.

How do family caregivers work to nurture the seeds of their insight? To begin with, it is important to understand that their insight has two aspects: its relationship to their ill family member *and* its relationship to themselves, personally.

Family members in the denial stage of their grieving process will often push to have their loved one returned to his or her previous environment – for example, back at school. Another common suggestion made by family members in denial is that their loved one, in order to get well, 'just needs a job.' As family members gain knowledge about their loved one's particular illness (its symptoms, treatments, prognosis, etc.) and learn, for example, that having people with mental illness return to school or work too soon is, in most cases, unsuccessful, they reconsider their suggestions and expectations.

Changes in expectation made in light of knowledge about illness *and* the particular struggle the loved one is experiencing with the illness, are clear signs of growth towards acceptance.

If you are a family caregiver, the other important aspect of developing and maintaining insight and acceptance involves a process of evaluating yourself and your role in caregiving. This means taking into account *your* personal reaction (that is, your grieving process) to having mental illness occur in your family. Looking at how you feel; how much time, energy, and money you have available; and how supported you are (morally and in practical ways) is critically important. Through consciously grieving how mental illness has changed your life, you can help yourself develop insight on a continual basis, both about yourself and your relationship with the person in your family who has illness. This is essential, in order to avoid dancing solely to the tune of your loved one's illness, and eventually burning out.

When you do make efforts to work at nurturing your insight about yourself in relationship to your loved one, you can also learn to give yourself permission to set limits on the care you give. For example, by putting limits on the amount of time, energy, and money you are willing to devote to him or her, you are at the same time *taking into account* and *respecting* your own needs. Make no mistake about it. This is something you must do to maintain your own physical and mental health.

SIGNPOST: Family members grieve individually

One further point family members benefit from knowing is this: *family members do not grieve in lockstep with each other.* This means, in part, that you most likely will have different views, both about the loved one's illness and about the relationships within your family (too dependent, over-protective, unsupportive). Often, the outcome is conflict within the family. Family conflict vis-à-vis the experience of mental illness is normal – not pleasant but *normal* nonetheless. Recognizing and expecting that you will have different points of view will help you be respectful of each other.

Here, I must again recommend that family caregivers join support and information groups. Your acceptance of the experience of mental illness in your family will be achieved and maintained only through deliberate efforts. To state the obvious, caring for a loved one who suffers mental illness can be difficult and sometimes *very* discouraging work. You need and deserve the support of a group, if for nothing else than to keep balance in your life so that your needs are also being met.

SIGNPOST: Acceptance requires activity

Acceptance is *not* a passive state! To come to any level of acceptance in relation to mental illness requires patient, continuous, and determined exercise, both mental and physical. We are *in process*, remember. And in the acceptance stage of grieving mental illness, we are, as we have been in the stages we have previously discussed, consciously choosing to be in tune with this process.

Just what activities are involved? Besides making efforts to keep our level of insight honed, we must also learn to continue to build and use coping skills. Of course, you have been building coping skills all along on your journey to recovery. For example, every time you focused to search for your feelings, or you gave yourself permission to cry, or you stared fear in its face, or you chose a constructive expression for anger, you exercised a coping skill.

An important first step in the acceptance stage is to ensure that you identify and claim the coping skills you have already built. Recognizing and owning your coping skills will allow you to consolidate and strengthen them, and will give you the confidence to go further and to build others.

When Barbara felt she had managed to grieve a severe bout of mental illness satisfactorily, she accepted my suggestion to take stock of what benefits she had gained through the experience. She waited about two weeks before giving her answer, but her reply showed that she had identified her coping skills and had recovered (or discovered) her sense of self:

As I think about what's happened to me over the last year, that is since I've consciously tried to heal from having had that attack, I can see that I've grown. I'm much more at ease with my emotional reactions. Now, if I feel like crying, I don't push this feeling away as if it were a feeling I shouldn't be feeling. I trust my feelings for what they can tell me about what's happening to me. And I now see that what is happening to me is something important.

Because I see myself this way now, I'm not always fighting with myself and devaluing myself. I'm at peace with the way I am. And also, when the company bosses tell us to take risks in our transactions, I don't shy away from risktaking as I always did before.

SIGNPOST: Affirmation is recovery's fuel

Affirmation means naming and claiming your personal growth and strengths, including all of the lessons you have learned through your struggle with mental illness. The acceptance stage of the recovery journey would be seriously deficient if affirmation of your experience and your growth – including your newly developed coping skills – were not affirmed, because one of affirmation's most important functions is to provide fuel for the continuing journey of recovery.

One of the best accounts of affirmation of personal coping know-how, and how it sometimes triggers support of others in the same boat, was made by a parent of a young man with chronic mental illness. He said:

> I have learned that sometimes I can cope with my grief about my son's illness only by acknowledging the good, for lack of a better word, I can do for someone else. When, for example, my son's condition was such that I could do nothing for him, to be able to pass on information learned from our experience to another parent was healing. In fact, doing this prompted me to look for more ways I might be of support to others in circumstances similar to ours.

I call that a sterling example of naming, claiming, and using coping skills!

Now that we have reviewed the three basic components of acceptance, we will turn our attention to some common issues and questions about acceptance.

SIGNPOST: Acceptance is an experience of one's own

Here, we will return briefly to a point made earlier, in order to emphasize the importance of realizing that each and every grieving journey, conscious or otherwise, belongs to an individual. Looking from the outside, others might and often do have good ideas about what the one they care about *should* be doing. Some examples:

'Joe shouldn't take medication.'

'Bertha should take medication.'

'Sharon should get retraining so she can get off welfare.'

'Stephen would do better if he'd move out of his parents' home.'

'Dora would do well to legally separate from him, or at least put him in a home and get on with her life.'

Unless people have been officially declared incapable of making decisions, their decisions are theirs to make.

Does this mean that caregivers should keep all their good ideas about various treatments and possible courses of action to themselves? Not at all. Coping with the experience of mental illness is not unlike other difficult tasks in life, and from time to time we will be in position both to give and receive 'good ideas.' But how each of us acts on the suggestions of others is our own decision to make.

SIGNPOST: You can deal with pressure from others with assertiveness

When pressure from others becomes a problem, and it cannot be avoided, consider an assertiveness training course.

Many people dismiss the idea of taking these courses because they believe that being assertive means being aggressive. They say they have no desire to become 'bossy.' Or (the more common explanation) that they already know how to put people 'in their place.'

These are wrong ideas about assertiveness. In my opinion, *the best* bet for dealing with pressure from others lies in assertiveness training. Learning its principles and skills helps us say what we want to say and gives us an understanding about the boundaries of our own power, and the power of others vis-à-vis ourselves. Assertiveness means, first of all, that I realize that where *I* stand as an individual has value, as does the position of the other person. Negotiating (having a balanced conversation with a goal in mind), *without losing face* and damaging self-esteem, can be a major pay-off of assertiveness training. (Just remember that, contrary to popular belief, assertiveness does not mean feeling free to tell the other guy off when you don't agree with him or her.)

SIGNPOST: Progress difficult or barely perceptible?

If you are like most of us, from time to time you will find yourself discouraged and perhaps exasperated with yourself, even at the acceptance segment of your journey. Maybe it is the task you have not completed or the goal you have set and not reached that is the problem. If this is so, I have two suggestions:

1. Adopt a *stance of patience* with respect to yourself. Yes, it will take effort, but it will make the acceptance segment of your recovery journey a little more comfortable. Feeling somewhat more comfortable, you can then pause to affirm the *progress you have made*, and to consider what you can do to have some additional successes in the near future.

2. Consider using the services of one of the growing number of professionals who are trained in psychiatric rehabilitation. These therapists work in collaboration *with* their clients so that developed goals are realistically achievable. They can also provide much needed coaching and support as you continue your trek to recovery.

SIGNPOST: Consider a psychiatric rehabilitation program

Formal psychiatric rehabilitation programs can offer a good deal of help, especially in areas related to activities of everyday living (for example, shopping, budgeting, cooking, housekeeping, working for money, and use of leisure time).

Coming to terms with or accepting one's psychiatric condition, whatever it is, makes for readiness to participate in the individual and group work that are part of rehabilitation programs. Complete acceptance is not necessary; only a willingness to work towards increased acceptance of one's psychiatric condition and towards your other goals.

SIGNPOST: Being human sometimes means failure

One of my high school teachers once told me to expect to fail 'not always, but sometimes.' This advice, spoken long before my encounter with mental illness, has helped me throughout my life to respect my efforts but not to see them as sure routes to success. As I have worked through my *conscious* recovery journey, this advice has redoubled in value. Expecting myself to fail 'not always, but sometimes,' has often helped me to accept myself as the fallible human I am.

I recommend my teacher's advice to you.

SIGNPOST: Professional caregivers are human, too

I have often heard from patients, families, and professional caregivers that one big difference between 'us' (professional caregivers) and 'them' (patients and family caregivers) is that we get to go home – that is, away from the scene of mental illness. This may be true in one sense. Yes, we can, for example, go home and expect to get a good night's sleep. As professional caregivers, we also get paid for what we do. But, in my opinion we do ourselves a great disservice if we do not take into account that, though we go home at the end of the day, *we do come back*. We come back *day after day* to help people who are dealing with very difficult problems.

Regardless of what we do in our leisure time, and how much training we have had to prepare ourselves for our work, most of us are challenged by our own sense of loss. Sometimes this sense of loss becomes particularly poignant when we see, again, someone in the throes of an acute phase of illness. Sometimes we notice a sense of loss within ourselves when we are with family members who are caring for someone who has a particularly severe type of mental illness. The question is how do we deal with our personal sense of loss?

It is encouraging to hear of professional caregivers openly grieving; for example, weeping along with family and friends at the scene of a patient's death. I believe, however, that generally, professional caregivers who work in a field of 'chronic loss' (such as mental illness, where problems often seem never-ending) often lose touch with their own sense of personal loss and their own need to grieve. I suggest two antidotes:

• recognizing that we as professional caregivers are human too, and that we also suffer loss in the face of the mental illness experience;

• grieving the personal loss in ways that are meaningful to us.

SIGNPOST: Still feeling sad, angry ... ?

One essential point to keep in mind, when we feel we have reached the acceptance segment of the recovery journey, is that the acceptance stage normally, and often, contains shades of the other stages of the grieving process. Awareness and recall of this reality keeps us from becoming alarmed when suddenly (or gradually) we feel, for example, bitter sadness, raging anger, or just plain discomfort about the presence of mental illness and its effect on our lives.

As we have seen throughout the conscious grieving process – when we are feeling our feelings of grief – *asking the key question is key!*

For myself, asking 'How can I help myself cope with my sadness about having been a patient in hospital for months at a time when my children were infants?' has helped me in many ways. I have been able to sharpen the focus of my feelings, to affirm *and feel* my feelings, and to decide when I am ready to let the feelings go – at least once again, and for now. I have had to ask key questions *many* times, and have had plenty of practice answering them. I know now that I have the coping skills to handle the return of grief feelings, and I know, too, that the feelings will continue to return.

My point in relating yet another of my own experiences in coping with the fallout of my mental illness experience is still the same: I want to give you a road map, one that I found both in studying what grieving experts have to say and by applying what I learned to my mental illness experience. To paraphrase what the grieving experts have to say to those of us whose lives have been touched with mental illness: *feel and use your grieving feelings and you will heal.*

The road map I have handed you is but a sketch. I hope that each of you, on your own recovery journeys, will complete this sketch in your own way, remembering that each of our journeys is unique.

SIGNPOST: Arriving at destination recovery

It is certain that the journey to the destination of recovery, like some other life journeys, does not have an exact ending point. We can get a sense that we have 'arrived.' Though illness may still be with us, we can feel more peace and a greater sense of confidence, or get in touch with long-lost aspects of ourselves. We can also expect to have shortcomings, but we will have learned ways of working with our healthy grieving process through to acceptance.

What is the password in acceptance? Simply, continuance. We must continue to ask and answer the key questions in order to find the answers we need.

Finally, my wish is that we patients and caregivers meet and support each other as we journey.

APPENDIX I

A Practitioner's Guide for Working with the Grief of Mental Illness

Grief is a subject that is not given much attention in most of our schools of professional training or in many of the agencies and institutions in which we work. As a result, it is not surprising that professional helpers often find themselves searching for appropriate ways to intervene when people who approach them are grieving.

Working with people and their grief when mental illness affects them or a member of their family poses special challenges. This is largely because this grief concerns a 'disenfranchised loss.'[1] In other words, it falls into a category of unrecognized loss. Consequences of the grief being unrecognized will be addressed in greater detail below.

In this appendix you will find a compact guide explaining how you can effectively work with your clients when they talk about the grief of their mental illness experience – or when they don't, but you think the time is right to address the constructive use of this process. Laid out in eight steps, the appendix contains key points with comments, as well as examples of dialogue between the worker and the person seeking help, to assist you to transport ideas on the pages of a book into your practice.

Step 1: Understanding the grief of mental illness process

There are two parts to understanding the grief of mental illness:

first, identifying the grief of mental illness as a grief process; and second, understanding the dynamics of normal grieving.

Chapter 1 of *Grieving Mental Illness* attempts to convey the importance of being able to recognize feelings of sadness, anger, or fear as grief reactions resulting from the mental illness experience so that one can do something with and about them. When attempting to raise the subject of these grief feelings, you might ask the person if he or she knows anything about working with the grief of mental illness. Once the conversation has started, your task is to explain that when people recognize difficult feelings they are at a point where they can work at alleviating these feelings. When people work at bringing themselves relief from burdensome feelings, they begin to notice not only a lightening in their mood but also a regained sense of control in their lives.

It is important that you assist the person to recognize that these feelings are part of a normal grieving process. If the grieving process is not understood as a normal, healthy, and healing process, it is likely that the grief experience will be wasted, endured without support, and, indeed, considered a problem or perhaps even part of the mental illness itself.

Whether working with an individual, family members, or a group, it is necessary to describe grief and its elements in detail – not only because people do not recognize their own grief, but even when they do, they often hold misguided notions about feelings of grief (e.g., 'I shouldn't cry'; 'It's a sin to be angry'). So the task of the worker is to teach key points about grieving, its process, and its dynamics, and then to facilitate conscious, constructive engagement in the process. You'll find some guidance for doing this in each chapter of *Grieving Mental Illness* and as outlined below.

Basic lessons about grief

- Denial, sadness, anger, and fear are all basic components of grief. They are not specific stages that an individual goes through only once. They can and do recur depending on a person's individual way of processing memories and external circumstances, e.g., anniversaries of loss, threats of various kinds – including the fear of another episode of illness.

- Each of the components can be present all at once.
- There can be a significant see-sawing effect between components of anger, sadness, shock, desperation, or fear. Some people, for example, find themselves sad one day, angry the next, and then feeling fear more than sadness or anger on the following day.
- The grief process is very personal and unique to each individual.
- There is no set norm for grief's duration. Grieving takes the time it takes.
- Grief is normal, healthy, and healing.
- Problematic grief can occur. This happens when, for example, people get stuck in a certain component of the process, somehow having sunk into an aspect of their grief process.

Workers need to pay attention to helping the person avoid a problematic grieving process. Understanding how problematic grieving comes about is therefore important. If there is a lack of awareness about the grieving process triggered by the mental illness experience and its many accompanying losses, people will not have a vision of grief's important component of 'acceptance.' In other words, they will have no idea of where they can get to psychologically and emotionally (e.g., enjoying regained feelings of peacefulness and confidence about themselves). Further, because of this lack of vision, they will be living without any hope of reaching acceptance and thus can remain unnecessarily stuck in their grieving process.[2]

Avoiding problematic grief in the case of mental illness is one of the reasons why there is great need for education and discussion about acceptance. But people also need to recognize the gains they've already made in grieving (and in other aspects of their lives), as well as further gains that can be made. At the very least, they need to know that their lives do not have to be constantly driven by whatever is happening with the illness. In other words, they deserve to know that they can get to a point where they feel that *they* – not the illness – are in charge of their lives.

It has been suggested to me several times that 'acceptance' could be better named. I agree. I have in fact found that discussions toward getting the right name for this component can be helpful in raising awareness about this component of grieving. Group participants have suggested other words and statements: '*accepting* – because we are talking about an *active* component of grieving and not a static phenomenon'; and '*integration* – because my illness has become a part of my life, a meaningful part of my life.'

In any case, I've found again and again that educational efforts focused on acceptance and the whole grieving process are facilitated if personal stories are told – stories of those who have successfully worked to come to terms with their mental illness experience. Storytelling exercises are, of course, greatly enhanced when told by the person who has struggled on his or her way to acceptance – or, if you like, 'accepting.'

Step 2: Listening to the person

As helping professionals, we are well aware of the critical role played by careful, active listening in getting a good picture of what the person before us is up against. It is a skill which not only helps us to avoid forming unfounded conclusions about the person's plight but also, and perhaps more importantly, serves to validate the person's experience. Throughout grief work the importance of listening to the person's story cannot be emphasized enough. Listening for the nuances in the story, asking for clarification and added detail, and using open-ended questions are the basics of adequate assessment as well as methods of conveying to the person our awareness and affirmation of their personal grief experience.

When listening to the person, monitoring the pacing of necessary interruptions (e.g., questions seeking clarification) is important. And when interruptions are in order, it is important to put these gently, indicating respect for the person who is speaking. For example:

'I don't mean to interrupt but it would help if I knew more about how that was for you.'

or

'Please excuse me for interrupting. I think I've missed something here. Would you mind reviewing that part for me again?'

Once we've taken the decisive step to listen for and to the grief expression of our clients, we have assumed a 'responsive position' for any expressions of grief as they come to the fore. Take, for example, expressions like:

'I'm sick of being sick!'

'I don't want to apply for disability – I want to get a job!'

'You're telling me that my son needs a supervised setting. I never dreamed that would be the case. Can't they make him better?'

If committed to being responsive, we will not be tempted to relentlessly continue with whatever task is at hand. We will instead turn to the person in their moment of grief expression, help them to put the finger on their grief, address it with them, and, then if at all possible, also complete the task at hand. In my practice, I've found that, on the whole, the moments I've taken away from tasks at hand to address expressions of grief have proven both to serve the person's 'in-the-moment' need for validation and to facilitate completion of the task at hand.

Step 3: Anticipating the grieving process

Once we have made the theoretical connection between the experience of mental illness and its attendant grieving process, we tend to notice in day-to-day practice that people experiencing mental illness encounter grief without recognizing it themselves. We know that some clients tend to be shy about talking about their personal lives. As well, when it comes to the grief experience, people can be reticent because they may not have the vocabulary to talk about it. It is likely they have not yet connected grief with the losses that accompany the experience of mental illness. Anticipating the grief reaction of the person is clearly of the essence.

Anticipating the grief response involves alerting people to what they can expect to have happen emotionally and psychologically because mental illness has touched their lives. This can be done by:

- asking the person how things are going for them personally
- listening for any connotations of grief in the response
- affirming the grief experience by talking further about it
- expanding on whatever points the person raises

Listening carefully to what John, in the following example, has to say regarding coping initiatives he has already employed is important. Affirming him in his coping efforts and raising his awareness – pre-emptively – about the part that fear, for example, plays in an overall grief process is also in order. As well, it might be a time to talk about the larger agenda of learning ways to arrive at acceptance.

> JOHN: Since my episode, I'm really afraid about never getting back to work – I mean, in a competitive job.
>
> WORKER: I hope you know about the vocational rehabilitation program at the clubhouse.
>
> JOHN: Yes, I've looked into that but I'm afraid I won't make it even with support. I feel stuck.
>
> WORKER: It sounds like you're encountering a component of grieving – grieving the experience of having to deal with episodes of psychosis. It's a process, you know. And, sometimes in this process people do feel stuck.
>
> JOHN: Well, I've sure got that feeling. I've got a feeling that I'll never make it out of this.
>
> WORKER: You are certainly showing signs of being able to take initiative again. For instance, you've looked into the clubhouse. Maybe I can help you understand your emotional process better so that you can learn to use that process toward your recovery and come to terms with your illness experience.

In summary, workers who have learned to anticipate grief are ready to respond appropriately when grief expressions come to the fore. As well, they can gently facilitate grief expressions from those who would not otherwise speak about it and provide affirmation of the person's efforts.

Step 4: Affirming the person along the course of the process

Efforts at conscious constructive grieving can be confounding. For example, once they become knowledgeable about some theoretical points about the benefit of actively grieving, some who suffer first-hand worry about becoming ill again if they go too far with the grieving process. Others – patients and family members – figure that once started on a 'grieving journey' they'll never be able to take another path, or as one mother put it, 'I might never stop crying if I start.'

As well as acknowledging perceptive questions and statements like these, it is important for the worker to affirm as normal any feelings of uncertainty the person might have about engaging with their grief. It might be helpful to liken first efforts on a grieving journey to the anticipation of a vacation or a trip to attend a family reunion. Fear of flying, concern about arriving at the correct destination, and nervousness about meeting old acquaintances and relatives we haven't seen in a long time are feelings most of us can easily relate to. By drawing comparisons like these, hesitations related to engaging consciously and constructively in the grieving process and its inherent component feelings are normalized, and the person receives a message of affirmation about wherever he or she is on the journey.

Gentle direction as to how to engage with one's own grief response can be conveyed when the question arises as to whether to take the plunge into the business of grieving. Alternatively, you can bring up the subject. Starting points should include guiding the person to:

• take notice of the feelings they are currently experiencing or have

experienced (that is, rather than digging for any which have not yet made themselves apparent)
- regard these feelings as normal and healthy
- explore feelings with a view to putting them to constructive use

Though the worker takes an educational role here as elsewhere in work with the grief of mental illness it's important to remember that, overall, the approach should be collaborative, taking into account the constructive coping skills the person is already employing. An example:

JENNY: Lately, I've been feeling lost. I know things have changed for me personally since the illness happened. I used to have my own business and because of illness I lost it. I thought I could have my own business again but now after the experience of trying but not having things turn out, I'm not so sure. I don't have the goals I once had and I don't know where to turn.

WORKER: It's important for you to know, Jenny, that your feeling of being lost is experienced by many people when illness becomes a part of their lives.

JENNY: Really?

WORKER: Yes, really. It sounds as if you are now very actively engaged in the process of coming to terms with the impact of your illness on yourself.

JENNY: Yes, and I know I need to accept my limitations.

WORKER: I trust you are looking at all the healthiness – all the capacity you still have – and also, though things have changed for you, that you have confidence that you will be able to find your way.

JENNY: I hope so. I do want to keep trying.

WORKER: What about changing your 'I'm lost' description of yourself to 'I'm trying to find my way'?

JENNY (after some pause): I think that would make a positive difference about the way I'm thinking about myself. I'd feel that I'm on my way in dealing with my illness and getting on to finding new goals.

WORKER: Right! New goals that are meaningful to *you*.

In working to affirm the person, the worker should take notice of unsuccessful ways of coping, including participation in destructive activities. Once addressed, unsuccessful ways of coping can be used as material for 'what we have learned for the next time' planning.

Acknowledging the need for taking breaks from the grieving journey is another affirmation task for the worker. The challenge of consciously and constructively grieving makes mandatory the need for periodic rest. People dealing with mental illness often need to be reminded of the importance of taking time out (e.g., taking a 'homemade Club Med') – and doing so without guilt – indeed, to honour themselves. Reminders such as 'No matter how hard life is, we still need to have the good times to keep us going!' help to drive home a message that dealing with mental illness is tough work and that breaks from it are as necessary as breaks from any kind of work.

Step 5: Passing on tools for constructive grieving

Along with deepening your own understanding of the grieving process, actively listening for expressions of grief, anticipating the grieving process, and offering your client purposeful affirmation, it is essential to pass on tools for the cultivation of grief. The two suggested most often in *Grieving Mental Illness* are the 'key coping questions':

'How can I help myself cope with <u>specific feeling / problem>?</u>'

and

'Is there anyway I can use my feeling of <u>anger / sadness / fear></u> constructively?'

These questions serve at least two purposes. They help the person first to focus on a particular, uncomfortable aspect of life and then to find ways to deal constructively with the problem. By using these questions on a routine basis, people report that they surmount slumps in mood and accompanying unproductive behaviour. The grief goes from being wasted to being useful.

The worker's task here includes introducing the key coping questions and then coaching the person in the use of these questions. In coaching, it's important to steer the person toward isolating a specific feeling or problem. Naming 'anger' as the problem is too general, but 'anger about the way my illness works' is workable because it is specific. After a specified focus is achieved, a problem-solving exercise can be employed to lead the person to personally meaningful and constructive answers to the key coping questions.

Examples of responses to the key coping questions about anger are:

'I know I've got a right to be angry about my illness.'

'I'm using the energy of my anger to work at and hang on to my recovery.'

'My anger can be turned into making things better for myself and for others I care about.'

At this point, coaching the person to hold the new insight and to put into practice a successful coping behaviour employed in the past or a new coping activity will serve to reinforce healthy insights about the grief experience. Inviting the person to try out a certain way of being or doing before you next meet is important. Once there is agreement on this, it is crucial that at the next meeting the worker inquire about how the new insight made a difference. (I find it helpful to jot a note in my agenda reminding me to ask.) Here again, careful listening and affirmation of any gains, or efforts toward gains, are in order not only to reinforce the person's endeavours but also to reinforce the use of specific coping tools, such as the key coping questions.

Both my group and individual work have taught me that the multitude of responses to the key coping questions – exercising, taking medication as prescribed, praying, taking a 'homemade Club Med,' cooperating with treatment, 'metathinking,' 'decentring,'[3] using the ABC model,[4] watching a tape that has helped before – though they may come slowly at first – come quite readily with practice and they unfailingly show sound, constructive insight.

You will find other examples of how the bits and pieces of grief expression can be put to constructive use in Chapters 2 to 7 of *Grieving Mental Illness*.

Step 6: Exercising a willingness to be with the person through the process

As a worker, being willing to be a companion to someone in their grieving process – wherever he or she is in the process – is essential. Grief expression has its ebbs and flows and will therefore be more intense at some times than at others. This does not mean that you need to be always available. First of all, that would be impossible, and second, you should not be the only support available to any one person. (I heartily agree with Mary Ellen Copeland's suggestion that each person needs a network of five supporters.)[5] It also doesn't mean that other tasks should be put aside indefinitely in order to focus on the person's grief work. Introducing notions about the benefits of setting long- and short-term real-life goals and working with the person toward achievement of these goals, all the while working with the grief, are what is necessary to foster recovery.

Step 7: Exploring 'guilt' and shame

As mentioned in Chapter 2, people who encounter mental illness experience of one kind or another often say they feel guilty. At our Family Information and Support Group meetings at the Royal Ottawa Hospital we have explored this feeling by first of all challenging it with the question, 'Guilty – for what?' As we delved into the subject for an answer – and gotten beyond (sometimes unhelpful) notions like 'survivor guilt' – constructive conclusions have been reached. One mother put it very well: 'I can now see that what I'd always called guilt – like the feeling I had when we'd go and enjoy a concert and my daughter didn't come – is really not guilt. It is profound sadness and frustration.' Naming feelings accurately is important because they then can be seen as normal and healthy, and as material for constructive use.

Another often-mentioned uncomfortable feeling is shame, and its close cousin, embarrassment. On exploration, workers find people are ashamed about all sorts of things that happen in the course of the mental illness experience: for example, police arriving at the door, bizarre and sometimes harmful behaviours, public disturbances, interruptions in career and academic pursuits, job loss. Workers need to assist the person to normalize feelings of shame. This is often accomplished by putting the shameful experience in the light of the 'big picture' of everything that has happened and is happening among us all on this planet. We can do this by asking questions like 'Who knows all the sides of the story of what happened anyway?' and 'How much exactly do you want to care about other people's opinions if they do know?' As well, shame can be alleviated by assisting the person to focus on the fact that he or she did survive the experience of job or career loss, of having the police present, or engaging in bizarre behaviour. Beyond this, assisting the person to focus on the source of their shame can be of help. Some useful questions can be:

- 'Who do you think is thinking about that incident right now?'
- 'If they are thinking about it, can you control what they are thinking?'
- 'How much do you think others are thinking of you and that incident?'
- 'How much of your life do you want to spend worrying about it?'
- 'Are you ready to let it go?'

In the face of an act that is indeed shameful (e.g., harm done to oneself or another), the worker can help by pointing out the power illness has in influencing the person to engage in unacceptable behaviour. This draws a useful and important distinction between the person and the illness. For those dealing first-hand with mental illness, this frame of mind puts them in a position of power – that is, both to manage the memory of that experience and to make future plans to avoid engagement in destructive activity.

Step 8: Feeling your own grief as a worker

There are several reasons for needing to feel your own grief as a worker. One of the most important is that you will remove any blight you might harbour of 'us versus them' thinking. As members of the human race, grief is part of our lot in life. As workers in the mental health field, we need to pay attention to the losses we experience in our work (that is, the losses we witness in the lives of others, which in turn render loss to us) and engage consciously and constructively in our grieving process. I believe that we are doing this as we sit listening to and commiserating with the person. These are meaningful steps in grieving – ones that lead us to know the feelings of powerlessness felt by the person in the face of illness and ones that, at the same time, can put us on a path to figuring out what the next constructive and meaningful steps ought to be. Allowing ourselves to experience our own feelings of grief also has the predictable effect of improving the way we practise. Glenn Bailley, a caregiver I met in Adelaide, Australia, at TheMHS 2000 Conference, puts it this way:

> An invaluable asset a worker or any fellow human being could have is the willingness to feel their own grief and as a result the compassion that it can engender. This is an asset for life and gives rise to one's ability to be with another's pain, grief or anguish, without deliberately creating a safeguard wall that impedes the ability to genuinely hear the other, verbally and emotionally.[6]

The eight steps outlined above are meant to give workers a brief but comprehensive course in working with the grief of mental illness. I hope that, in coming to a clearer understanding of the grief of mental illness and how to work with it, workers will find that many benefits accrue. In particular, I hope you, as workers, notice a boost in your empathy level as well as a broadening of your choices of therapeutic approaches and methods as you set out to assist the person who is on a recovery journey – a very precious time for both of you.

102   Appendix I

NOTES

1 For detail about disenfranchised loss, see K.J. Doka, *Disenfranchised Grief: Recognizing Hidden Sorrow* (Lexington, MA.: Lexington Books, 1989) and V.R. Pine et al. (eds.), *Unrecognized and Unsanctioned Grief: The Nature and Counseling of Unacknowledged Loss* (Springfield, Ill.: Charles C. Thomas, 1990).

2 For greater detail, see V. Lafond, 'The Grief of Mental Illness: Context for the Cognitive Therapy of Schizophrenia,' in C. Perris and P.D. McGorry (eds.), *Cognitive Psychotherapy of Psychotic and Personality Disorders: Handbook of Theory and Practice* (Chichester: John Wiley & Sons, 1998).

3 Metathinking and decentring are cognitive behavioural therapy techniques cited by Carlo Perris in *Cognitive Therapy with Schizophrenia Patients* (New York: Guilford Press, 1989).

4 The ABC Model, a cognitive behavioural therapy technique, is outlined in P. Chadwick, M. Birchwood, and P. Trower, *Cognitive Therapy for Delusions, Voices and Paranoia* (Chichester: John Wiley & Sons, 1996).

5 M.E. Copeland, *Creating Wellness: Key Concepts for Mental Health* (video tape). Available from the Mental Illness Education Project, Inc. P.O. Box 470813. Brookline Village, MA 02447; www.miepvideos.org.

6 G. Bailley, 'Painting a Picture of the Unrecognized Grief of Mental Illness' (unpublished paper).

APPENDIX II

*Grieving Mental Illness: Responses to Frequently Asked Questions**

It has been fifteen years since I first began working with concepts of grief as they relate to the mental illness experience. Over these years, as I have focused on this subject and attempted to spread the word about the benefits of engaging actively in this grieving process, questions have arisen from all sectors – from people affected first-hand by mental illness, from family caregivers and friends, and from professional and volunteer helpers. For some time, I've realized I owe a debt of gratitude to everyone who participated in discussions with me and particularly to those who asked questions. The questions stand out in my mind as touchstones, for they greatly assisted me to refine my ideas about both the grief of mental illness and working with that grief. More than anything else, they fostered the development of what I believe is a sensible and sensitive approach to this work.

This appendix lists the questions most frequently asked, along with responses I've developed about the grief of mental illness and about working with it. They are listed here in no particular order of their frequency or importance.

* The material in this appendix is an elaboration of my keynote address delivered at the 10th Annual TheMHS Conference of Australia and New Zealand, August 2000.

Question 1: Is there a basis in the literature for the grief of mental illness?

Yes, there is. When I attempted my first literature searches, looking for material about assisting patients with the psychological and emotional consequences of mental illness, I found little to draw upon. I did find some acknowledgments and descriptions of the presence of grief – or other reactions which could be considered 'grief-like' – related to the mental illness experience.[1] Few of these were developed to any extent and certainly not to the point where they could be easily carried into a therapist's practice, and thus eventually be of practical use to people affected.[2] However, they were helpful to me as far as they went, and certainly – because they did only go so far – they provided much of the inspiration for writing *Grieving Mental Illness*.

I've had many opportunities to speak publicly on the subject of grief and mental illness since the book's publication in 1994, and thanks to these opportunities, I've continued to be both a teacher and a student of the grief of mental illness. This student-teacher stance has led to more discoveries in the literature – both in the stories told by people affected and in the professional literature. I have found both sources to be equally helpful in my endeavours to understand the grief of mental illness and its potential for healing.

The stories that people tell of their mental illness experience, whether they are affected directly or as families members, unfailingly speak about the experience of the grief of mental illness. They illustrate grief's dynamic within the individual as well as its spill-over into the person's social network. The following snippets from four of the many stories I've come across are good examples.

Margo Button, a Canadian poet, dedicated her first published book of poetry, *The Unhinging of Wings*,[3] to her late son, Randall John Button, who ended his life by suicide in 1994. The following is an excerpt from her poem 'Family Tree':

In the summer of '92   I return to the family home
Stumps remain of the four old elms

that framed the white farmhouse   Here
in the barnyard I made mud pies with pee
when I was two   Sweet grasses buzz and blow
in the sun where Dad ran with his brothers
and sister Anna   the aunt I resemble

Only Dad and his brother remain
of Bartlett's whose photos once covered the wall
We eat lobster sandwiches at Grandpa's oak table
Uncle talks about the folks down the road
who had a son an only son   They locked him
in the barn when he had a crazy spell

I imagine fists pounding splintery wood
until they bled in the black where the voices were
Fists in my chest   *My son Randall John*
I tell them   *is mentally ill*
The cause is genetic   The prognosis is not good
I want to add *I regret I cannot replace him*
but I will not let him disappear

Dad twists his mouth and scowls at the sideboard
He wishes I hadn't brought it up   Uncle studies
the crusts on his plate   This family of men know
only the touch of handshakes   They talk easily
about the price of shingles at the sawmill or the deer
whose soft white bellies they slit in the fall   Pain
they pour down their gullets and piss out in the drain   (pp. 44–5)

Anne Deveson, in her book *Tell Me I'm Here,*[4] has several
acknowledgments and descriptions of her own and others' grief
relating to her son's mental illness. Her journal/diary entry of 22
January 1981, for example, reads:

At the end of the afternoon I was driving through North Adelaide
when I spotted him walking along the middle of the road. He waved
at me to stop. He asked me for a milkshake so we went into a cafe,

and talked for a few minutes before he began glowering at me, and
muttering ...

One minute Jonathan was blowing into his chocolate-malted. The
next, he had thrown the milkshake at my face, followed by the pepper and salt, upturned the table, and chucked a chair at me. People
gasped, the waiter came running and Jonathan shot off, out the door
and up the street. I shook the milk off me and tried to rub the pepper
out of my eyes, which made it worse ...

Brenda and Margaret thought I should charge Jonathan with
assault. They said I had to set limits. The idea appalled me. But I did
feel angry: angry with Jonathan for hurting me, angry with the system for not helping him, angry with the illness. The hardest anger to
deal with was the anger with Jonathan, because of its paradox. Can
you be angry with someone if it is their illness that makes them so
destructive? But I *was* angry, so angry that I felt like thumping anyone and everyone, so angry that I had to belt my rage out on some
cushion, and even then could not assuage it because I felt so power-
less. (p. 82)

Another writer, who has suffered mental illness first-hand and
who writes from the viewpoints of both 'consumer' and professional is Julie Leibrich, Mental Health Commissioner in Welling-
ton, New Zealand. In *A Gift of Stories: Discovering How to Deal
with Mental Illness*[5] she shows herself not only to be a quintessen-
tial gatherer of stories but also one who has generously told her
own story. Her grief, as she opens her story, cannot be mistaken.
She writes:

My life has been enormously influenced by episodes of depression.
They took away years of my life as a young woman. They influenced
the *path* of my life for twenty years. They were the reason I didn't
have a family until it was too late to do so. I lost homes. I lost a husband. I lost friends. I lost many things I otherwise might have had.
(p. 173)

Stewart D. Govig is an American Lutheran minister, the father of
a son with schizophrenia, and the author of *Souls Are Made of*

Endurance: Surviving Mental Illness in the Family.[6] At one point in his book, he describes a time when he and his wife attempted to strictly follow professional advice, specifically, to enforce their expectations of their son – in this case, for him to arrive home at a reasonable hour. His grief expression is here patent.

> We would keep the doors locked at night. Yet in the cold darkness, to keep the door closed before the solitary, unshaven and dishevelled figure standing in the porch light meant anguish difficult to describe. It went against what I think must be one of the deepest instincts of any parent. To have provision and power but refuse it to your own child is a fierce test of endurance. How often Ann and I *almost* opened that front door.
>
> He slept in the lawn equipment shed a few nights and then asked a favor: Could he hitch a ride downtown? Nearing our destination, he asked to stop for a 'treat' ... Afterward no words were exchanged as he picked up his meagre belongings and headed out into the night. On his own, he would have to find a 'mission' or church-run shelter. Alcoholics and addicts would be the roommates; bright college kids were now a curious thing of the past.
>
> On the way back toward our warm and comfortable suburban home, the splashing of windshield wipers kept time with the flooding waves of my sadness. Even if someone had thought to ask how Jay was doing, what would I have said? (p. 46–7)

The Professional Literature:

Although still limited, the professional literature focusing on the grief of mental illness is beginning to have more and more to tell us. It can be grouped roughly into two main categories. One contains research findings which are testament to the presence of grief in family members.[7] The second comprises descriptions of grief as it plays out in the lives of those who are affected by mental illness first-hand.[8] In both categories, it is usual to find suggestions for practitioners to develop awareness and sensitivity about the dynamic of the grieving process among individuals and family members.

In addition, the literature which examines the phenomenon of grief in general (that is, not specifically related to mental illness) has been of help in my work with the grief of mental illness. For example, certain questions, such as whether grief and its various aspects should be considered as normal emotion or as pathological process,[9] have caused me to look at whether there is not a great deal of unresolved grief in the case of mental illness, especially because the losses related to mental illness fall into the category of disenfranchised or unrecognized grief.

Another category is the literature which challenges the assumptions of some grief and trauma theories and their various spin-offs into therapeutic approaches.[10] This critical body of literature serves to inform and reform mental health practice. Conclusions, for example, that someone's grieving has gone on 'far too long' (evolving sometimes into unhelpful injunctions like 'Get away from your grief!' or 'You've got to move on!') are put under scrutiny by critical thinkers and researchers. We are helped through their work not only to avoid making mistakes in our grief work, but also to develop approaches which genuinely serve those we try to serve.

Question 2. Where's the connection between work with the grief of mental illness and cognitive behavioural therapy?

Cognitive behavioural therapy (CBT) is a reason-based treatment approach designed to help people resolve their personal psychological and behavioural problems. One of the hallmarks of CBT is that the therapist teaches the person to use techniques or tools for managing various symptoms or problems which crop up from time to time. CBT is not a therapy that is 'done to' the person but rather 'done with' the person. Typically, once the therapist has outlined ways and means of using CBT tools, the therapist's role becomes that of a coach and an affirming companion on the recovery journey. At this point, therapy sessions can be scheduled at greater intervals and later there will be need for booster sessions only.

To my mind, work with the grief of mental illness provides both a theoretical framework and a practical context for CBT. As well, it offers some 'tools of the trade' for CBT. I have elsewhere outlined in detail my reasoning for proposing grief work as the context for CBT.[11] This proposal that the grief of mental illness be considered as a context for CBT took shape as I noticed from my CBT practice (and other work as well) that people often change whatever subject is at hand to express grief. In these moments, I began to recognize that whenever the person and I have a task at hand – for example, a CBT exercise to control paranoia – and the person suddenly blurts out 'I'm just so tired of all this!' or 'My bills are mounting up. I wish I could work at a real paying job like I used to!,' it is not the time to insist that we carry on through the metathinking exercise. It is, rather, time for working with the person's current emotional presentation, returning to the task at hand once the person's grief distress has been alleviated.

I have used and found success with the 'key coping questions,' as proposed in *Grieving Mental Illness*, over the course of my group work practice with patients who have serious mental illness. The practice of asking, and responding to, the questions 'How can I help myself cope with <u><feeling / specific problem></u>?' and 'Is there any way I can use my <u><anger / sadness / fear *constructively*></u>?' sharpens the cognitive focus and guides the person behaviourally in a positive way. In other words, in consciously and constructively using these tools to work with the grief experience through the use of the key coping questions, the person is on a path of thinking and behaving that generates healing, personal meaning, and a desire to make the world a better place.

The benefit of using these questions as CBT tools in a group setting usually becomes quickly apparent. With minimal coaching, participants focus on their 'coping success stories,' as well as their not-so-successful attempts at coping (along with the lessons learned), and move towards ways of dealing with their current issues. Group participants often benefit from the stories told by others. One group participant's words echo those of many others: 'I thought I was the only one with ideas like mine until I came to the Coping with Illness Group. I went through five years of torture because I thought I was in a class by myself. Now I don't feel so alone, and also I've learned how to handle my painful thinking.'

Question 3: Should the notion of work with the grief of mental illness be introduced in 'early phase' work? If so, how and when should it be introduced?

Thankfully, the last decade has seen an increase in efforts worldwide to comprehensively treat young people who present with signs of mental illness. Many benefits have already accrued. For example, 'early phase' work in schizophrenia means that schizophrenia is no longer viewed as it once was – a progressively debilitating illness with increasingly serious symptoms. Rather, it is viewed as a serious but treatable illness.[12] Treatment involves medication, support, and education – including education about the condition and presenting symptoms, about prescribed medication, about what to expect and how problems and symptoms can be managed. It is important to note that education is offered not only to the person affected first-hand but also to family members.

To be sure, the young person who encounters psychosis is faced with its enormous challenges. The question, 'Is it necessary to introduce the subject of grief and grief work as part of the person's education, given that the person already has enough to deal with?' is certainly a fair one.

After giving this question a great deal of thought, my answer is yes. My reasoning is grounded in a sense of professional responsibility arising from my observation of grief expression in young people who suffer 'first episodes' of psychosis, as well as from documentation based on research studies.[13] Thus my conclusion: To leave any person who is suffering early phase or later phase psychosis, without the knowledge about a process she or he will in all likelihood experience – and without training in ways of dealing with this process – is to short-change the person.

Introducing ideas about the grief of mental illness and working with it can be done in individual or group context, and is probably more effective if delivered in both. The therapist should choose when, what, and how much information to dispense, depending on both the presenting needs of the young person and his or her current ability to receive new information. Therapists often need to find wording other than 'grief' or 'grief reaction' especially when we know these words won't fit for the person. Asking questions such as 'How are you coming to terms with this experience?' and 'What do you make of your personal experience with a psychiatric problem?' can lead the young person to a new level of emotional and psychological awareness vis-à-vis the trauma of their illness experience and provide, at the same time, a valuable opportunity for information about the grieving process.

Those of us who facilitate groups for young adults know well that we often find moments within sessions which are perfect for inserting a purposeful message about the importance of learning about coming to terms with mental illness, including psychotic experiences. I call these 'teaching-off-the-topic moments.' Sometimes, of course, it is best not to derail the subject at hand for the group as a whole by attending to an individual's grieving process. Adept group facilitation does demand attention to the group as a whole as well as to the needs of individual participants. Taking a moment to convey a word of direction to an individual (e.g., that you will meet after the group session about whatever grief issue he or she has just expressed) fosters the group's current focus, and, at the same time, recognizes and validates – for all participants – the individual's grief expression.

Question 4: Is the grief of mental illness a metaphor or a literal phenomenon?

'Grief? Why grief?... Why have you connected grief and mental illness? ... You've got the wrong metaphor!' After more than a decade of working to develop concepts about work with the grief of mental illness, I still find myself stopped in my tracks when I hear questions and remarks like these. I stammer, wondering if the person has two minutes, two hours, or two weeks to engage in conversation with me, or even time to read a book on the subject.

I am aware that there is a line of thinking among some professional caregivers that we should not be introducing what they would call 'negative' topics, like grieving, and that instead we should be focused on conveying hope through 'positive' messages. With due respect, I say that such an approach shows the marks of professional and personal denial of the grieving process that occurs with mental illness and, because it does, it falls short of serving people's needs adequately.

In answering the question, 'Is the grief of mental illness a metaphor or a literal phenomenon?,' perhaps it would be better to ask, 'Is grief a metaphor – that is, any more than words are metaphors for conveying what happens in life?' In other words, does the word 'grief' adequately capture the emotional process that occurs as a result of the mental illness experience?

To avoid simplistic wordplay and to get on with the task of answering this question, I have found the wisdom of Berger and Luckman helpful. They point out that 'language is capable not only of constructing symbols that are highly abstracted from everyday experience, but also of "bringing back" these symbols and [presenting] them as objectively real elements in everyday life.'[14] As one who makes it part of my professional business to advance a message about 'the grief of mental illness,' I take from Berger and Luckman a strong word of warning that I had better be sure that I am calling the human experiences I think are ones of grief by the right name. After much study, observation, listening, and thought, I have concluded that grief is the right name for the anguish we go through in the wake of mental illness.

Question 5: Would it be better to approach the emotional and psychological consequences of mental illness with a trauma model rather than a grief model?

This is an excellent question, containing as it does ideas for a conversation or indeed a debate about the best approach to assist people with the consequences of their mental illness experience. At this point, the literature gives no indication which approach would be most useful.

In any event, I believe it would be counterproductive to get into polarized positions about the use of either a grief model or a trauma model. Why not both? As McGorry et al. point out, disastrous events, including mental illness, 'give rise to a range of sequelae *including loss and trauma.*'[15]

Ultimately, what is important is that the person be given tools to manage the psychological experience accompanying the mental illness experience, with emphasis on two equally important goals: (1) coming to meaningful and peaceful terms about the experience, and (2) relapse prevention.

Question 6: Can the model you've developed for working with the grief of mental illness be applied to other grief and trauma experiences?

A friend, recently widowed, called me to thank me for writing *Grieving Mental Illness* because 'though I set out to read it to know what it contained as I was giving it to my sister who has two children who suffer from schizophrenia, I found it to be a journey for me – a way to come to terms with Jim's death.' My friend's words reminded me of the advice of other friends and colleagues. Many have suggested that I should write more on grief as it occurs in various life circumstances, using the approach as outlined in *Grieving Mental Illness*. I'll always remember the enthusiasm of one social work colleague in particular when she remarked, 'The grief model in your book can be used to help people grieving anything – trauma, alcoholism, death of a loved one, death of a pet, divorce.' I agree.

The heart of the work within *Grieving Mental Illness* is the recognition of the grieving process and the constructive use of that process in order to come to peace about the losses involved in the mental illness experience. I do believe people can use the two key coping questions ('How can I help myself cope with <u>this particular problem / feeling ></u>?' and 'Is there any way I can use the energy of my <u><sadness / anger / fear / frustration> </u>constructively?') and find help to deal with their grief in most, if not all, of life's tough circumstances. These circumstances would, for example, include the threats of war and terrorism, and their accompanying losses of safety and security, in the wake of the events of September 11, 2001.

Catastrophic events, like those that occurred on September 11, involve a series of serious losses, including loss of life, material losses, and loss of peace of mind. In the wake of these losses, we recognize that we often behave differently – so differently that we can find ourselves on occasion wondering if, in our measures to take precautions, we are overreacting. In all circumstances of loss, it is important to remind ourselves that the grieving process is, first of all, a normal process and, also, that it is an individual process – ideally, supported by the community which might also be sharing the loss – and that most of us will do what we must to come to terms with our losses. And, yes, it can be helpful to have a guide, as proposed in *Grieving Mental Illness,* to engage constructively in the process.

NOTES

1 V. Lafond, 'The Grief of Mental Illness: Context for the Cognitive Therapy of Schizophrenia,' in C. Perris and P. McGorry (eds.), *Cognitive Psychotherapy of Psychotic and Personality Disorders: Handbook of Theory and Practice* (Chichester: John Wiley, 1998).
2 One particularly helpful exception is J.J. Jeffries, 'The trauma of being psychotic,' *Canadian Psychiatric Association Journal* (1977): 22.
3 M. Button, *The Unhinging of Wings* (Lantzville, BC: Oolichan Press, 1996).
4 A. Deveson, *Tell Me I'm Here* (Victoria, Australia: Penguin Books, 1992).
5 J. Leibrich, 'Discovering the Life You Want,' in *A Gift of Stories: Discovering How to Deal with Mental Illness* (New Zealand: University of Otago Press, 1999).
6 S.D. Govig, *Souls Are Made of Endurance: Surviving Mental Illness in the Family* (Louisville: Westminster John Knox Press, 1994).
7 See, e.g., F. Miller, J. Dworkin, M. Ward, and D. Baron, 'A Preliminary Study of Unresolved Grief in Families of Seriously Mentally Ill Patients, *Hospital & Community Psychiatry* 41 (12 Dec.): 1321–5; G.G. Eakes, 'Chronic Sorrow: The Lived Experience of Parents of Chronically Mentally Ill Individuals, *Archives of Psychiatric Nursing*, 9/2 (1995): 77–84; P. Solomon and J. Draine, 'Examination of Grief among Family Members of Individuals with Serious and Persistent Mental Illness,'

Psychiatric Quarterly, 67/3 (Fall, 1996): 221–3; P. Solomon, J. Draine, E. Mannion, and M. Meisel, 'Effectiveness of Two Models of Brief Family Education: Retention of Gains by Family Members of Adults with Serious Mental Illness, *American Journal of Orthopsychiatry,* 67/2 (Apr. 1997): 177–86; D.J. Davis and C.L. Schultz, 'Grief, Parenting, and Schizophrenia,' *Social Science & Medicine,* 46/3 (Feb. 1998): 369–79.

8 See, e.g., M.A. Selzer, T.B. Sullivan, M. Carsky, and K.G. Terkelsen, *Working with the Person with Schizophrenia: The Treatment Alliance* (New York: New York University Press, 1989); M.T. Appelo, C.J. Sloof, F.M.J. Woonings, J. Carson, and J.W. Louwerens, 'Grief: Its Significance for Rehabilitation in Schizophrenia, *Clinical Psychology and Psychotherapy* 1(1), 53–9; V. Lafond, 'The Grief of Mental Illness: Context for the Cognitive Therapy of Schizophrenia,' in C. Perris and P. McGorry, (eds.), *Cognitive Psychotherapy of Psychotic and Personality Disorders: Handbook of Theory and Practice* (Chichester: John Wiley, 1998); P. MacGregor, 'Grief: The Unrecognized Parental Response to Mental Illness in a Child, *Social Work* 32/2 (Mar. 1994): 160–6.

9 See, e.g., M. Viederman, 'Grief: Normal and Pathological Variants, *American Journal of Psychiatry,* 152/1 (Jan. 1995): 1–4.

10 See, e.g., J.R. Averill and E.P. Nunley, 'Grief as an Emotion and as a Disease: A Social-Constructionist Perspective, *Journal of Social Issues,* 44/3 (Fall, 1988): 79–95; C.B. Wortman and R.C. Silver, 'The Myths of Coping with Loss, *Journal of Consulting and Clinical Psychology,* 57/3 (June 1989): 349–57; H.G. Prigerson, E. Frank, S.V. Kasl, C.F. Reynolds III, B. Anderson, G.S. Zubenko, P.R. Houck, C.J. George, and D.J. Kupfer, 'Complicated Grief and Bereavement-Related Depression as Distinct Disorder: Preliminary Empirical Validation in Elderly Bereaved Spouses, *American Journal of Psychiatry,* 152/1 (Jan. 1995): 22–30; D. Summerfield, 'War and Mental Health: A Brief Overview, *British Journal of Psychiatry,* 152/1 (Jan. 2000): 1–4.

11 Lafond, 'The Grief of Mental Illness.'

12 Schizophrenia Society of Canada, *Learning about Schizophrenia: Rays of Hope; A Reference Manual for Families and Caregivers* (Toronto: Schizophrenia Society of Canada): 15.

13 As noted in the response to Question 1. Though I recognize that these

studies are not specific to early phase work, they indicate the need for grief work regardless of the particular phase of mental illness.

14 P.L. Berger and T. Luckman, *The Social Construction of Reality: A Treatise in the Sociology of Knowledge* (Garden City: Doubleday, 1962): 40.

15 P.D. McGorry, L. Henry, D. Maude, and L. Phillips, 'Preventively-Oriented Psychological Intervention in Early Psychosis,' in Perris and McGorry, eds. (1998): 221 (emphasis added).

Bibliography

Ambrose, Joann. (1989) 'Joining In: Therapeutic Groups for Chronic Patients'. *Journal of Psychosocial Nursing. 27*, (11).

Anderson, Robert, & Bury, Michael. (1988) *The Experience of Patients and Their Families. London: Unwin Hyman.*

Beck, A., Rush, A., Shaw, B., & Emery, G. (1979) *Cognitive Therapy of Depression.* New York: Guilford Press.

Buckman, Robert. (1992) *How To Break Bad News: A Guide for Health Care Professionals.* Toronto: University of Toronto Press.

Butler, Pamela E. (1991) *Talking to Yourself: Learning the Language of Self-Affirmation.* San Francisco: Harper.

Davidson, Glen W. (1984) *Understanding Mourning: A Guide for Those Who Grieve.* Minneapolis: Augsburg Publishing House.

Dearth, Nona et al. (1986) *Families Helping Families: Living with Schizophrenia.* New York: W.W. Norton.

Deegan, Patricia E. (1988) 'Recovery: The Lived Experience of Rehabilitation'. *Psychosocial Rehabilitation Journal, 11*, (4).

– 'How to Integrate and Involve Consumers in All Levels of the Mental Health System.' An Address to the Ottawa-Carleton Branch of the Canadian Mental Health Association Conference, Feb. 21, 1991.

Dershimer, Richard. (1990) *Counseling the Bereaved.* New York: Pergamon Press.

Deveson, Anne. (1992) *Tell Me I'm Here.* Victoria, Australia: Penguin Books.

Dincin, Jerry. (1990) 'Speaking Out.' *Psychosocial Rehabilitation Journal, 14*, (2).

Dinner, Sherry. (1989) *Nothing to be Ashamed Of: Growing Up with Mental Illness in Your Family.* New York: Lothrop, Lee & Shepard Books.

Doka, Kenneth J. (1989) *Disenfranchised Grief: Recognizing Hidden Sorrow.* Lexington, MA.: Lexington Books.

Endler, Norman. (1982) *Holiday of Darkness.* New York/Toronto: John Wiley & Sons.

Farkas, Marianne D., & Anthony, William A. (1989) (Eds.) *Psychiatric Rehabilitation Programs: Putting Theory into Practice.* Baltimore: Johns Hopkins University Press.

Fieve, Ronald R. *Moodswing.* (1975) Toronto: Bantam Books.

Gendlin, Eugene T. (1982) *Focusing.* Toronto: Bantam Books.

Gunderson, John G. (1978) 'Defining the Therapeutic Processes in Psychiatric Milieus.' *Psychiatry, 41.*

Harris, M., & Bergman, H.C. (1984) 'The Young Adult Chronic Patient: Affective Responses to Treatment.' In B. Pepper & H. Ryglewicz (Eds.), *Advances in Treating the Young Adult Chronic Patient.* San Francisco: Jossey-Bass.

Hatfield, Agnes, & Lefley, Harriet P. (1987) (Eds.) *Families of the Mentally Ill: Coping and Adaptation.* New York: Guilford Press.

Health and Welfare Canada. (1991) *Schizophrenia: A Handbook for Families.*

Hughes, Gerard W. (1985) *God of Surprises.* London: Darton, Longman & Todd Ltd.

Jeffers, Susan. (1987) *Feel the Fear and Do It Anyway.* New York: Fawcett Columbine.

Jeffries, J.J. (1977) 'The Trauma of Being Psychotic.' *Canadian Psychiatric Association Journal, 22.*

Johnson, Julie Tallard. (1988) *Hidden Victims: An Eight-Stage Healing Process for Families and Friends of the Mentally Ill.* New York: Doubleday.

Kanter, Joel S. (1985) (Ed.) Clinical Issues in Treating the Chronically Mentally Ill. In New Directions for Mental Health Services, 27. San Francisco: Jossey-Bass Inc.

Kübler-Ross, Elisabeth. (1969) *On Death and Dying.* London: Tavistock.

Kurelek, William. (1982) *Someone With Me: The Autobiography of William Kurelek.* Toronto: McClelland & Stewart.

Lagrand, Louis E. (1988) *Changing Patterns of Human Existence: Assumptions, Beliefs, and Coping with the Stress of Change*. Springfield, Ill.: Charles C. Thomas.

Lerner, Harriet Goldhor. (1985) *The Dance of Anger: A Woman's Guide to Changing the Patterns of Intimate Relationships*. New York: Harper & Row.

Levine, Helen. (1982) 'The Personal Is Political: Feminism and the Helping Professions.' in *Feminism in Canada: From Pressure To Politics*. Finn, Geraldine, & Miles, Angela (Eds.). Montreal: Black Rose Books.

Lindemann, E. (1944) 'Symptomatology and Management of Acute Grief.' *American Journal of Psychiatry, 101* (2).

Littlewood, Jane. (1992) *Aspects of Grief: Bereavement in Adult Life*. London and New York: Tavistock/Routledge.

McMullin, Rian E. (1986) *Handbook of Cognitive Therapy Techniques*. New York, London: W.W. Norton.

Menninger, Karl; Mayman, Martin; & Pruyser, Paul. (1972) *The Vital Balance: The Life Process in Mental Health and Illness*. New York: Viking Press.

Mercato, Sharon. (1992) The Shell People: My Story of Schizophrenia. Brampton, Ont.: Ashlar House Publishing & Promotions.

Mohelsky, Helmut. (1987) 'The Functionalist Approach to Psychiatric Rehabilitation.' *Psychosocial Rehabilitation Journal, X*, (4).

Parkes, Colin Murray. (1972) *Bereavement: Studies of Grief in Adult Life*. New York: International Universities Press.

– (1986) *Bereavement: Studies of Grief in Adult Life* (rev. ed.). London: Penguin Books.

Parkes, Colin Murray, & Weiss, Robert S. (1983) *Recovery from Bereavement*. New York: Basic Books.

Perris, Carlo. (1989) *Cognitive Therapy with Schizophrenic Patients*. New York: Guilford Press

Pine, Vanderlyn R.; Margolis, Otto S.; Doka, Kenneth; Kutscher, Austin H.; Schaefer, Daniel J.; Siegel, Mary-Ellen; & Cherico, Daniel J. (Eds.). (1990) *Unrecognized and Unsanctioned Grief: The Nature and Counseling of Unacknowledged Loss*. Springfield, Ill.: Charles C. Thomas.

Rando, Therese A. (1984) *Grief, Dying, and Death: Clinical Interventions For Caregivers*. Champaign, Ill.: Research Press Company.

– (1986) *Loss and Anticipatory Grief*. Lexington, MA.: Lexington Books.

Raphael, Beverley. (1983) *The Anatomy of Bereavement*. New York: Basic Books.

Sanders, Catherine M. (1992) *Surviving Grief ... and Learning to Live Again*. New York: John Wiley & Sons, Inc.

Sederer, Lloyd (Ed.). (1983) *The Therapeutic Milieu in Inpatient Psychiatry: Diagnosis and Treatment*. Baltimore: Williams and Williams.

Seeman, M.V. et al. (1982) *Living and Working with Schizophrenia*. Toronto: University of Toronto Press.

Siris, Samuel G. (1991) 'Diagnosis of Secondary Depression in Schizophrenia: Implications for DSM-IV.' *Schizophrenia Bulletin, 17*, (1).

Staudacher, Carol. (1991) *Men and Grief: A Guide for Men Surviving the Death of a Loved One*: A Resource for Caregivers and Mental Health Professionals. Oakland, CA: New Harbinger Publications.

Strauss, John S. (1992) 'The Person-Key to Understanding Mental Illness: Towards a New Dynamic Psychiatry, III.' *British Journal of Psychiatry, 161* (18), 19–26.

Styron, William. (1990) *Darkness Visible: A Memoir of Madness*. New York: Random House.

Torrey, E. Fuller. (1988) *Surviving Schizophrenia: A Family Manual* (rev. ed.). New York: Harper & Row.

Vash, Carolyn L. (1981) The Psychology of Disability. New York: Springer Publishing Co.

Viorst, Judith. (1986) *Necessary Losses*. New York: Simon and Schuster.

Wasserman, Harry, & Danforth, Holly E. (1988) *The Human Bond: Support Groups and Mutual Aid*. New York: Springer Publishing.

Wechler, James et al. (1988) *In a Darkness: A Story of Young Suicide*. Miami: Pickering Press.

Worden, J. William. (1982) *Grief Counseling and Grief Therapy: A Handbook for the Mental Health Practitioner*. New York: Springer Publishing.

Index